Glossary

Actinic keratosis (solar keratosis): a sun-induced, precancerous, cutaneous lesion, presenting as a scaly patch or plaque, comprising atypical keratinocytes microscopically

5-ALA: 5-aminolevulinic acid – a naturally occurring substance in the human body that is converted to protoporphyrin IX, a photosensitizer, especially in actively growing cells; often present in precancers or cancers

Basal cell carcinoma (BCC): a low-grade skin cancer; the most common human malignancy, composed microscopically of basaloid cells, which are locally invasive and rarely metastasize

Bowen's disease: a scaly, erythematous plaque that is a type of in-situ squamous cell carcinoma

Breslow thickness: cutaneous melanoma thickness, measured histologically from the top of the viable epidermis (granular layer) to the deepest tumor cell in the skin; an important prognostic indicator

Broders' histological grade: classification system for squamous cell carcinoma in which grades 1, 2 and 3 denote ratios of differentiated to undifferentiated cells of 3:1, 1:1 and 1:3, respectively; grade 4 denotes tumor cells with no tendency towards differentiation

Chondrodermatitis nodularis helicis: a small, benign but painful papule on the helix of the ear caused by inflammation of the ear cartilage

Clark's level of invasion: a grading system for the level of invasion of primary cutaneous melanoma in which level I is confined to the epidermis, level II extends to the papillary dermis past the basement membrane, level III fills the papillary dermis and compresses the reticular dermis, level IV invades the reticular dermis and level V involves subcutaneous tissue. Like Breslow thickness, it correlates with risk of metastasis, with a worse prognosis for the higher levels

Cryosurgery: a dermatologic treatment in which a very cold substance or cryogen (usually liquid nitrogen) is applied to the skin to freeze cutaneous lesions and cause controlled necrosis

Dermatoscope: a handheld magnifying instrument that assists with the examination of cutaneous lesions

Epidermolysis bullosa dystrophica: an inherited blistering disease, characterized by atrophy of blistered areas, severe scarring and nail changes that occur after separation of the epidermis

Erythema ab igne: a red-brown hyperpigmentation of the skin caused by chronic local exposure to heat

Erythroplasia of Queyrat: squamous cell carcinoma in situ of the glans penis

Gorlin's syndrome: an inherited disease in which a mutated gene (*PTCH*) predisposes to development of tens to hundreds of BCC and to certain other developmental anomalies

Hedgehog signaling pathway: a cascade of signaling molecules that influence embryologic development and later cell division, in which mutations can lead to BCC and other malignancies

HPV: human papillomavirus, responsible for warts; only certain subtypes are related to the development of cancer

Hyperkeratosis: thickening of the outer layer of skin

In situ: in place – a cancer that has not spread to invade neighboring tissues

Keratinocyte: a cell of the epidermis characterized by keratin production

Keratoacanthoma: a rapidly growing epidermal tumor comprising well-differentiated atypical keratinocytes; the tumor usually regresses spontaneously; more aggressive forms are often difficult to differentiate from squamous cell carcinoma

Lentigo (plural: lentigines): a dark spot with more pigment cells than normal skin; a sign of sun damage but lacking malignant potential

Lentigo maligna (Hutchinson's melanotic freckle): an irregularly pigmented macule most commonly found on the face and/or neck of older people representing in-situ melanoma with the potential to progress into invasive malignant melanoma (lentigo maligna melanoma)

MAL: methyl aminolevulinate – used as a photosensitizer in photodynamic therapy

Mammillated: having nipple-like projections

Melanocyte: a melanin-producing cell situated in the basal layer of the epidermis; the normal counterpart of a melanoma cell

Melanoma: a cutaneous tumor with strong metastatic potential, comprising malignant melanocytes

Mohs' micrographic surgery: a procedure in which a cutaneous neoplasm is excised and the margins frozen-sectioned and assessed histologically in stages as the tumor is removed; the wound is only repaired when there is histological confirmation of complete excision

Nevomelanocyte: precursor of a melanocytic nevus cell derived from either epidermal melanoblasts or dermal Schwann cells

Nevus: developmental abnormality. A melanocytic nevus (commonly a mole); a cluster of benign pigment cells that usually appear in the first decades of life ('bathing trunk' nevi are congenital lesions that cover a large area of the body)

Parakeratosis: retention of nuclei in the upper layers of the epidermis

Photodynamic therapy (PDT): a treatment in which a photosensitizer such as 5-ALA or MAL is applied to the tissue and then activated by a source of visible light, resulting in cell destruction

Punch biopsy: a small skin specimen for histological assessment obtained by using a circular blade attached to a handle

PUVA: administration of psoralen (a phototoxic drug), which acts as a skin sensitizer, followed by exposure to ultraviolet A (UVA) light; used to treat psoriasis, vitiligo and other skin diseases

Seborrheic keratosis: a benign, pigmented, often papillomatous cutaneous lesion generally seen in older individuals; also called stucco keratosis

Squamous cell carcinoma (SCC): a malignant cutaneous neoplasm, derived from keratinocytes, that usually presents as an enlarging nodule on sun-exposed sites; these tumors have metastatic potential

Sunburn cells: keratinocytes undergoing apoptosis as a result of ultraviolet irradiation

Sun protection factor (SPF): a number that quantifies the degree of protection given by a sunscreen from the erythemogenic wavelengths (primarily UVB). The SPF value is obtained by dividing the exposure time required to develop barely detectable erythema (sunburn) for sunscreen-protected skin by that for unprotected skin

UV: ultraviolet; the portion of sunlight energy responsible for sunburn, tanning and cancer

Xeroderma pigmentosum: a rare autosomal-recessive disorder of defective DNA repair characterized by more than a thousandfold risk of UV-induced skin cancer

Introduction

Skin cancer is important to doctors, both generalists and specialists, and to the public because it is common (and becoming more so), preventable and treatable.

There are three main types: malignant melanoma and the two non-melanoma skin cancers, basal cell carcinoma (BCC) and squamous cell carcinoma (SCC). Well over a million people in the USA and about 100 000 in the UK develop a skin cancer each year. Most of these cancers are BCC, and many of the affected people will have, or have had, at least one other skin cancer.

Twenty years ago, melanoma was the 27th most common cancer in the USA, but it is now the seventh, and it has become the most common solid tumor in adults. Melanoma, particularly, and SCC can kill – there are about 7500 deaths from melanoma in the USA each year and about 1800 in the UK, more than double the figures of 20 years ago.

In part, our current problems with skin cancer are the result of mass emigration from northern Europe over the last two centuries, with fair-skinned people settling in sunnier climes such as North America, Australia, New Zealand and South Africa. Climate change, longevity, recreation and hedonism are important additional factors.

Skin cancer is caused by damage to DNA from ultraviolet (UV) light combined with failure to repair that damage effectively and/or failure to eliminate or repair precancerous skin lesions.

Theoretically, skin cancer can be prevented by educating people about, for example, recreation, clothing, sunscreens and sunbeds (primary prevention), but this approach could take a generation or more before it has a sizeable effect. Serious morbidity and mortality can be prevented or reduced (secondary prevention) by educating patients and physicians alike, so that at-risk individuals and early lesions are identified with accuracy. In Australia, the 5-year survival of patients with melanoma increased to 85% by the year 2000, from around 50% in 1980.

Surgery is usually the treatment of choice, although there are other options, mainly for precancerous situations such as actinic (solar) keratoses. The increasing volume of skin-cancer work has implications for the planning of medical staffing levels and healthcare delivery systems. Although relatively simple surgery suffices for most cancers in most patients, some require multidisciplinary input (dermatologist, plastic surgeon, radiotherapist and oncologist).

National and international consensus guidelines have evolved, and these assist practice (especially by non-experts), education, training, audit and research. Mohs' micrographic surgery has resulted in significantly improved cure rates for selected skin cancers, particularly BCC. Unfortunately, effective treatment of disseminated disease, which has a high mortality, remains difficult. The management of advanced melanoma, for example, consumes a very high proportion of the overall budget for the disease.

Although the incidence of skin cancer is growing rapidly worldwide, most malignancies are treatable if they are diagnosed early enough. With this in mind, we aim to present the basic facts about the epidemiology, causation, presentation and management of skin cancer in an easily accessible way, and we hope that *Fast Facts – Skin Cancer* will be of interest and value to a wide readership. We have included key references throughout the book to support the principal points and to facilitate further inquiry.

Basal cell carcinoma

Basal cell carcinoma (BCC) is the most common malignant neoplasm in white populations. Its incidence has increased in recent decades: the highest rates are in Australia, where it affects over 2% of men. The tumor most commonly arises on the head and neck (Figure 1.1) and, overall, the incidence is higher in men than in women.

Risk factors. The risk of BCC is increased in those who:
- have a history of severe childhood sunburn(s)
- have red hair
- tan poorly.

The association with sunlight is not well understood. Cumulative ultraviolet (UV) exposure was conventionally thought to be the most important risk factor. However, exposure to the sun during childhood and adolescence and, particularly, intense intermittent exposure may be of greater importance than previously thought in the development of BCC.

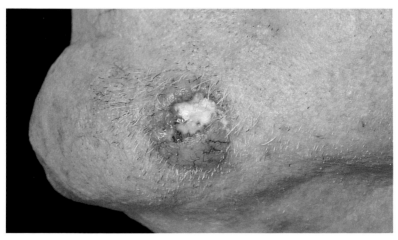

Figure 1.1 BCC most commonly arises on the head and neck.

Other risk factors for BCC include:
- North European ancestry
- a positive family history
- immunosuppression
- exposure to arsenic
- previous radiotherapy.

BCC can develop in a sebaceous nevus (Figure 1.2). It is also associated with a number of conditions, including albinism, xeroderma pigmentosum (a rare autosomal-recessive disorder that affects DNA repair), nevoid BCC syndrome (Gorlin's syndrome) and human immunodeficiency virus (HIV) infection.

Table 1.1 summarizes the risk factors for BCC compared with squamous cell carcinoma and melanoma.

Squamous cell carcinoma

Cutaneous squamous cell carcinoma (SCC) is the second most common skin cancer in white populations; SCC represents roughly 20% of all non-melanoma skin carcinomas. The incidence of non-melanoma skin cancer (BCC and SCC together) is approximately 18–20-fold greater than that of melanoma.

SCC is most commonly seen in the elderly and is three times more common in men than women. The incidence is rising, being

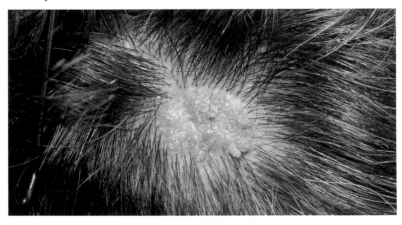

Figure 1.2 Sebaceous nevus on scalp – BCC and SCC can develop from this type of birthmark.

TABLE 1.1

Risk factors for skin cancer

	Basal cell carcinoma	Squamous cell carcinoma	Melanoma
Sex	Male > female	Male > female	Male > female
Age	Middle-aged to younger	Older	Younger
Relationship to sun exposure	Childhood; intermittent	Chronic	Childhood; intermittent
Sunburn history	Severe sunburn in childhood	Episode of severe sunburn	Episode of severe sunburn
Tanning ability	Non-tanners	Non-tanners	Non-tanners
Skin color	Fair skin/freckles	Fair skin/freckles	Fair skin/freckles
Hair color	Red	Red/blond	Red/blond
Eye color	Not documented	Not documented	Blue
Precursor lesions	Actinic keratosis	Actinic keratosis	Nevi

highest in countries with high sun exposure. In 1994, SCC accounted for 2500 deaths in the USA; the incidence of SCC was thought to be between 24 and 59 per 100 000 women and between 81 and 136 per 100 000 men.

Lesions occur on sun-exposed sites, predominantly the head and neck (Figure 1.3).

Risk factors. UV radiation is the strongest etiologic factor. In particular, sun exposure, both recent and cumulative, is implicated in SCC development. This malignancy is more common in fair-skinned individuals with red or blond hair (see Table 1.1).

The acquired risk factors for SCC include:
- a history of severe sunburn
- sunbed use

- 200+ treatments with psoralen and UVA phototherapy (PUVA) (e.g. for psoriasis)
- chronic immunosuppression (e.g. as occurs with alcoholism, HIV infection, chronic lymphatic leukemia and organ transplantation).

Much of the research identifying the association between immunosuppression and SCC has been performed in the organ transplant population. The risk of developing SCC is increased in organ transplant recipients, and the ratio of BCC to SCC incidence is reversed in this population.

Other predisposing factors for SCC include previous exposure to polycyclic hydrocarbons or radiation (Figure 1.4), exposure to arsenic and infection with the human papillomavirus (HPV). Further genetic risk factors include conditions with *p53* gene mutation, xeroderma pigmentosum and albinism.

In addition, invasive SCC is recognized to develop from actinic keratosis and in-situ SCC, as well as at sites of chronic injury, such as ulceration, infection, scars and epidermolysis bullosa dystrophica (a condition characterized by atrophy of blistered areas and severe scarring).

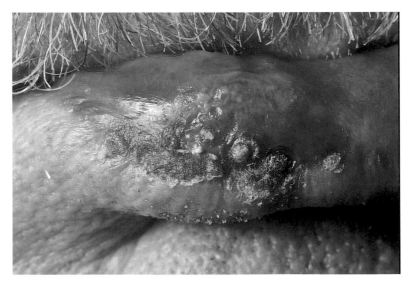

Figure 1.3 SCC on the lip – these lesions predominantly occur on sun-exposed sites, particularly the head and neck.

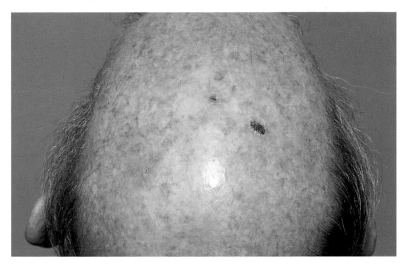

Figure 1.4 Radiotherapy-damaged scalp on which a SCC subsequently developed.

Melanoma

The incidence of melanoma is increasing faster than that of any other human cancer. It primarily affects white-skinned people, in whom the incidence increases with age and is inversely related to the latitude of residence. Melanoma occurs more commonly in men, and mortality is higher in men, particularly in those aged over 50. It is most commonly found on the limbs of white women and the faces or backs of white men (Figure 1.5).

Plantar and subungual melanomas are very rare, but when melanoma develops at these sites it is seen most often in black populations and people from south east Asia and the Indian subcontinent.

Internationally, the incidence of melanoma varies: there are approximately 40 melanomas per 100 000 people per annum in Queensland, Australia, and 10 per 100 000 in Germany and the UK. Fortunately, the survival rates are improving as the proportion of thin melanoma (≤ 0.75 mm) being diagnosed is increasing. In New South Wales, Australia, the overall 5-year survival rate for melanoma was 50% in 1980, whereas in 2000 it had improved to 85%.

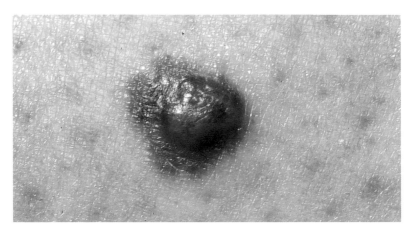

Figure 1.5 Nodular melanoma, with Breslow thickness 1.8 mm.

Risk factors. The development of superficial spreading and nodular melanoma correlates more with exposure to intermittent intense sunlight than with chronic UV exposure. The risk of melanoma (see Table 1.1) increases in people with:
- fair complexions
- freckles
- blue eyes
- red or blond hair.
  Other predisposing factors include:
- an increased number of normal (Figure 1.6) or atypical nevi
- a history of severe sunburn during childhood or adolescence
- an inability to tan.

A positive family history is also a risk factor, predominantly as a consequence of predisposing family traits. The term familial malignant melanoma is used when two or more first-degree relatives develop melanoma. These individuals tend to develop multiple thinner melanomas, and the age at onset is lower than in the general population. Familial malignant melanoma accounts for 5–12% of all melanoma; only a small subset of affected individuals are likely to have an inherited melanoma susceptibility gene mutation. Predisposing genes have been identified, one of which is also identified with pancreatic cancer (this is covered briefly in Chapter 2, Pathogenesis).

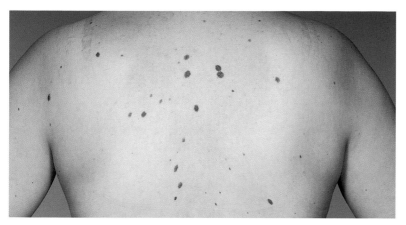

Figure 1.6 Multiple nevi – a risk factor for melanoma.

Other risk factors for malignant melanoma include:

- iatrogenic immunosuppression
- PUVA treatment (e.g. for psoriasis)
- xeroderma pigmentosum
- HIV infection
- atypical nevus syndrome (see page 38).

Malignant melanoma can develop from congenital or acquired melanocytic nevi. The risk is highest in congenital melanocytic nevi that have a diameter greater than 20 cm, and is as high as 15% in giant 'bathing trunk' lesions – congenital lesions that cover large areas of the body.

Key points – epidemiology

- Deaths from skin cancer continue to rise.
- Ultraviolet exposure is the most important risk factor.
- Early diagnosis saves lives.

Key references

Bagheri MM, Safai B. Cutaneous
malignancies of keratinocytic origin.
Clin Dermatol 2001;19:244–52.

Bunker CB, Gotch F. AIDS and the
skin. In: Burns T, Breathnach S, Cox
N, Griffiths C, eds. *Rook's Textbook
of Dermatology*, 7th edn. Oxford:
Blackwell Science, 2004: 26.1–26.41.

Diepgen TL, Mahler VM. The
epidemiology of skin cancer. *Br J
Dermatol* 2002;146(suppl 61):1–6.

Gallagher RP, Hill GB, Bajdik CD
et al. Sunlight exposure, pigmentary
factors, and risk of nonmelanocytic
skin cancer. I. Basal cell carcinoma.
Arch Dermatol 1995;131:157–63.

Gallagher RP, Hill GB, Bajdik CD
et al. Sunlight exposure,
pigmentation factors, and risk of
nonmelanocytic skin cancer. II.
Squamous cell carcinoma. *Arch
Dermatol* 1995;131:164–9.

Goldman GD. Squamous cell cancer:
a practical approach. *Semin Cutan
Med Surg* 1998;17:80–95.

Goldstein AM, Tucker MA.
Genetic epidemiology of cutaneous
melanoma: a global perspective.
Arch Dermatol 2001;137:1493–6.

Lang PG Jr. Malignant melanoma.
Med Clin North Am 1998;82:
1325–58.

Lear JT, Harvey I, de Berker D et al.
Basal cell carcinoma. *J R Soc Med*
1998;91:585–8.

Roest MAB, Keane FM, Agnew K
et al. Multiple squamous skin
carcinomas following excess sunbed
use. *J R Soc Med* 2001;94:636–7.

Skidmore RA Jr, Flowers FP.
Nonmelanoma skin cancer. *Med Clin
North Am* 1998;82:1309–23.

Stern RS. PUVA follow up study. The
risk of melanoma in association with
long-term exposure to PUVA. *J Am
Acad Dermatol* 2001;44:755–61.

Stern RS, Lunder EJ. Risk of
squamous cell carcinoma and
methoxsalen (psoralen) and UV-A
radiation (PUVA). A meta-analysis.
Arch Dermatol 1998;134:1582–5.

Basis of malignancy

Integrity of the genome is critical to life. Even one miscoded or incorrectly expressed protein can have catastrophic results. In higher organisms such as man, disturbing the exquisite balance between growth and differentiation of cells in a way that leads to cancer is a relatively common and sometimes lethal error.

In many tissues, including skin, it is absolutely necessary for cells to divide throughout life. The outer layer is continuously shed and must be replaced by terminally differentiating cells generated from the layers just below. If cell division and differentiation fail, infection and electrolyte loss can rapidly lead to death. Yet too much cell division, coupled with impaired differentiation, constitutes a malignant tumor. The excess cells can also migrate elsewhere (metastasis), divide in other parts of the body and severely impair organ function.

Oncogenes. Many decades ago, researchers discovered that infection with certain viruses caused malignant tumors in animals. They then found that specific viral genes, termed oncogenes or cancer-causing genes, encoded proteins that caused uncontrolled growth of infected cells. Normal mammalian cells were found to contain very similar or identical genes that functioned or 'turned on' in response to specific signals to stimulate cell division; mutated gene products (proteins) could be permanently 'turned on', like the viral oncogenes, leading to continuous inappropriate cell division or cancer. The normal, unmutated versions of such genes are now termed proto-oncogenes, implying that they can be converted to oncogenes. A common example is *RAS*. Mutations in such genes are usually dominant, that is, if only one of the cell's two copies is mutated, the result is abnormal proliferation.

Tumor suppressor genes. A second group of genes that contributes to cancer was discovered in children at high risk of retinoblastoma.

Affected children often lost both eyes to these malignant retinal growths and, if they survived, often died of a third malignancy in another organ. These children were found to have a mutation in one copy of the retinoblastoma gene of which the protein product (pRb) served as a critical 'brake' on cell growth, especially in certain cell types. If the second normal copy of the gene was inactivated for any reason, the affected cells would begin to divide uncontrollably. Further research revealed many such tumor suppressor genes and cancer-prone syndromes, in which one gene copy is abnormal from birth (or, in most cases, from conception) and a later random mutation of the second copy leads to malignancy. In families strongly predisposed to dysplastic nevi and melanoma, the inherited mutation is usually in the *CDKN4A* gene that encodes two tumor suppressor proteins, p16INK4a and p14ARF. Mutations in this gene also predispose family members to other malignancies, notably pancreatic carcinoma.

Perhaps the best known is *p53*, also known as 'the guardian of the genome', a transcription factor and DNA-repair protein that is dysfunctional in half of all human malignancies. It is now clear that loss of function of the tumor suppressor gene is extremely common in spontaneous malignancies, despite the requirement for both copies of the gene to be compromised, a statistically rare event. This is strong testimony to the important role of tumor suppressor proteins in modulating normal cell growth.

Carcinogens. Cancer develops as a result of cumulative DNA damage, most often due to a combination of carcinogen exposure and genetic vulnerability. UV radiation (sun exposure) is the most important contributory factor for skin cancer, but in some individuals exposure to other carcinogens, such as cigarette smoke or chewing tobacco, arsenic or therapeutic X-irradiation, may also contribute.

A classic early example of skin cancer due to carcinogen exposure was the development of otherwise rare scrotal cancers in chimney sweeps in England caused by the chemicals present in soot, which penetrated through their clothes and into this vulnerable area of skin.

Effect of age. The incidence of all skin cancers rises exponentially with age, due in part to the opportunity for cumulative mutations over time. Vulnerability to new damage also appears to increase with age, in part because of decreased expression of DNA-repair proteins.

Photocarcinogenesis

The role of UV radiation is twofold:

- damage to the DNA, causing mutations in the genes that regulate cell growth, including proto-oncogenes and tumor suppressor genes
- an immunosuppressive effect on the skin.

UVB radiation is more photocarcinogenic than UVA, photon for photon, but UVA is far more abundant in sunlight. It is likely that both contribute to the development of skin cancer.

When UV photons are absorbed by DNA, photoproducts or distorted linkages form. The most common is the dimeric fusion product of two adjacent DNA pyrimidine bases (Figure 2.1). The predominant photoproduct, accounting for up to 85% of DNA lesions after UV radiation, is the cyclobutane pyrimidine dimer. If not properly repaired, the photoproduct can lead to a point mutation in the DNA, because DNA polymerase is unable to interpret the altered bases and inserts the wrong 'partner' in the new complementary DNA strand that it synthesizes (Figure 2.2). Fortunately, before DNA synthesis occurs, the photoproducts are usually repaired by nucleotide-excision-repair enzymes, which avert tumor formation. However, there is evidence that this capacity to repair DNA declines with age, leading to an increased risk of unrepaired mutations.

UV radiation also induces cutaneous immunosuppression, which favors tumor survival, because lymphocytes otherwise appear capable of destroying malignant cells by recognizing the new proteins (antigens) they often express on their surface. The mechanism of UV-induced immunosuppression, which has been extensively studied in mice, is not completely understood. However, sunlight causes cells to release immunosuppressive chemicals or cytokines and alters the antigen-presenting function of Langerhans cells. It may also play a role in the generation of suppressor versus helper T lymphocytes that prevent other lymphocytes from destroying 'foreign' cells.

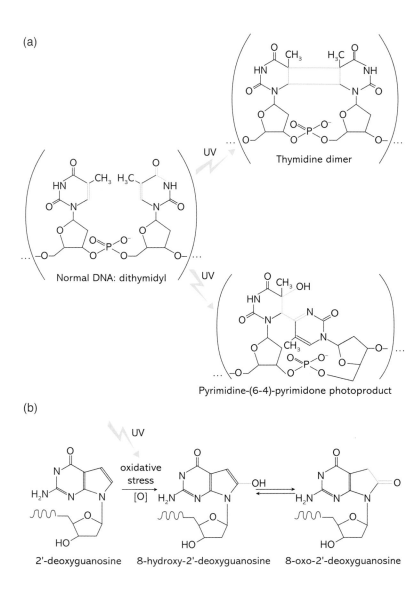

(a)

Thymidine dimer

Normal DNA: dithymidyl

UV

UV

Pyrimidine-(6-4)-pyrimidone photoproduct

(b)

UV

oxidative
stress
[O]

2'-deoxyguanosine   8-hydroxy-2'-deoxyguanosine   8-oxo-2'-deoxyguanosine

Figure 2.1 UV-induced DNA damage. (a) UV photons may be absorbed directly
by DNA, leading to new covalent bonds between adjacent pyrimidines. Both
cyclobutane pyrimidine dimers (more common) and (6-4)-pyrimidine–pyrimidone
photoproducts may be formed. (b) Both UVB and UVA can also damage DNA by
producing free radicals that in turn oxidize DNA bases, usually guanine. If
unrepaired, either type of damage can lead to a DNA point mutation.

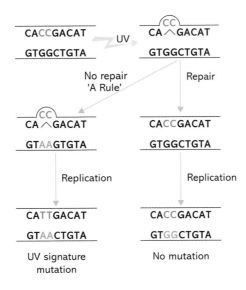

Figure 2.2 UV signature mutations. No carcinogen other than ultraviolet (UV) radiation produces pyrimidine photoproducts. In contrast, many carcinogens and even normal cellular metabolism, in addition to UV, can cause damage to other DNA bases, especially guanine (G). The most characteristic signature mutation is CC → TT: when unable to 'read' bases properly during DNA replication, DNA polymerase uses the 'A rule' and places adenine (A) opposite the distorted unreadable base(s). If a dimer consists of TT, placing the AA on the newly synthesized complementary strand results in no change in sequence because AA is the normal complement to TT. Hence, no mutation. In the above diagram of an arbitrary gene sequence, however, an unrepaired UV-induced CC dimer results in AA on the new complementary strand. This, in turn, dictates TT, not CC, during the next round of DNA replication. Hence, a mutation. C → T is also considered a change likely to have been caused by UV, for the same reason. In contrast, a damaged G paired with A by DNA polymerase will give rise to a non-specific G → T mutation.

Genetic predisposition

Most (perhaps all) tumors result from DNA mutations in the genes responsible for regulating cellular growth or DNA repair. Multiple genetic lesions in a single cell are usually required before its unregulated growth gives rise to a solid tumor.

There are a number of recognized genetic mutations that are associated with cutaneous malignancies.

p53 is a tumor suppressor gene (as discussed above) that influences many cellular functions, including cell cycle arrest, programmed cell death, cellular differentiation and DNA repair. It is also a transcription factor, and as such can increase or decrease production of other gene products. The encoded *p53* phosphoprotein senses DNA injury and arrests cell division to provide time for DNA repair; if the DNA damage is severe, *p53* induces cell apoptosis. UV-induced *p53* gene mutations are seen in nearly all SCCs and approximately 50% of BCCs. *p53* mutations are also common in sun-damaged skin, premalignant actinic keratoses and Bowen's disease. This suggests that loss of *p53* function occurs early in the stepwise progression from a completely normal epidermal cell to a frankly malignant one, probably because the loss of *p53* function makes it easier for cells to accumulate other mutations.

Xeroderma pigmentosum. Patients with this rare disease have a mutation in one of the genes that encodes the proteins involved in nucleotide excision repair, required for removal of UV-induced DNA damage. When DNA damage in growth-regulating genes is not repaired, tumors can arise. Skin cancers begin to develop in the first decade and often lead to death in the patient's teenage years or twenties. This can only be prevented by complete protection from the sun, starting in infancy.

PTCH. The *patched* (*PTCH*) gene is another tumor suppressor gene. It has a central role in the so-called hedgehog signaling pathway that stimulates growth. In autosomal-dominant nevoid BCC syndrome (Gorlin's syndrome), one copy of *PTCH* is mutated and inactive in all body cells. As for pRb and retinoblastoma discussed above, if the second gene copy is lost in a single cell it begins to divide excessively and a tumor develops. Patients with Gorlin's syndrome often have hundreds of BCCs that start to arise in adolescence. *PTCH* mutations are also common in sporadic BCC.

RAS. The *RAS* family of proto-oncogenes encodes G proteins that are involved in growth-factor signaling. *RAS* mutations have been found in cutaneous melanoma, SCC and actinic keratosis.

p16. Inherited *p16* gene mutations have been identified in some relatives of people who have a genetic predisposition for melanoma. Many sporadic melanomas are also found to have mutations or loss of expression of this tumor suppressor gene, known to act in the same signaling pathway as pRb.

MC1R. Another genetic predisposition to skin cancer involves the melanocortin-1 receptor (*MC1R*), the cell-surface receptor for α-melanocyte-stimulating hormone (α-MSH). Although originally named for their roles in stimulating pigment production in skin and hair, these proteins are now also known to influence immune function and possibly even DNA repair. Variants of the normal *MC1R* gene sequence are common in humans, and some less active variants have been strongly linked to fair freckled skin and red or blond hair, as well as to a high risk of skin cancer, including melanoma. The receptor encoded by these variants is not considered mutant, but it signals far less well than the normal receptor after binding with α-MSH, and is likely to contribute directly to the predisposition for cancer, at the very least by compromising protective melanin production. Such variations among key proteins still considered to be within the 'normal' range almost certainly contribute to cancer predisposition in the skin and indeed in all organ systems as observed in the general population.

Other predisposing factors

In addition to the specific gene mutations described above, viral infections have been shown to affect the pathogenesis of SCC. Particular strains of human papillomavirus (HPV) have high oncogenic potential and have been implicated in the development of in-situ and invasive SCC. Here, viral DNA is incorporated into the host genome, influencing cell differentiation and growth. Viral genes that inactivate *p53* have been studied in detail.

Immunocompromised individuals – for example, organ transplant recipients or those with HIV infection – have an increased risk of non-melanoma skin cancer. It is presumed that dysplastic keratinocytes are not identified or are not eradicated effectively by immune surveillance, and malignancies are more likely to develop.

Relationship to pattern of UV exposure

Cutaneous melanoma arises from epidermal melanocytes, whereas SCC and BCC develop from keratinocytes. Although UV exposure plays a major role for all three malignancies, their statistically associated patterns of exposure are different. Melanoma is associated with intense intermittent exposure to sunlight, and it most commonly develops on sites of the body that receive UV intermittently. In contrast, SCC is associated with chronic cumulative sun exposure. This type of malignancy tends to occur in people with substantial daily sun exposure, such as farmers or sailors, and in habitually maximally sun-exposed sites.

The reason for these differences is unknown, but recent insights into how cells respond to UV exposure allow for speculation. The melanocytes produce melanin and distribute it to surrounding keratinocytes. Melanin is hence able to absorb UV photons that might otherwise damage DNA or cell membranes and is photoprotective. When skin is irradiated with sunlight, melanin production increases, as does the capacity for cellular DNA repair. It is thought that skin cells are therefore most vulnerable to UV radiation after prolonged periods of sun avoidance, when the melanin content and DNA-repair capacity are low. In addition, melanocytes are more resistant to UV-induced apoptosis than keratinocytes and hence more likely to survive highly damaging exposures and undergo mutations as a result. Perhaps, for these combined reasons, intermittent UV radiation is more important in the development of melanoma than of SCC; that is, unlike the melanocyte, the keratinocyte is unlikely to survive high-dose radiation, but recurrent low-dose UV radiation may gradually allow mutated clones to develop. Basal cells, the least differentiated of the epidermal keratinocytes, are likely to have a resistance to apoptosis intermediate between that of melanocytes and the suprabasilar keratinocytes from which SCC develop. This level of resistance would explain the epidemiological association of BCC with intermittent UV exposure as well as with chronic UV exposure.

Key points – pathogenesis

- Cells have many cancer-prevention mechanisms. Usually, several of them must be impaired in a single cell before uncontrolled (malignant) growth ensues.
- Cells lose anticancer defenses through mutation or decreased expression of the responsible gene products.
- Cancers usually contain a combination of mutations in proto-oncogenes (which create an oncogene and continuous positive-growth signaling) and in tumor suppressor genes (which disable the cellular 'brakes' or negative-growth signaling).
- Very rarely, mutations occur spontaneously. Far more often they result from exposure to DNA-damaging agents, also called carcinogens.
- Heritable disorders with a high risk of skin cancers are the result of mutations in the germline that either reduce DNA-repair capacity or compromise one of the important growth regulatory pathways in the cell.
- For skin, the major carcinogen is ultraviolet irradiation.

Key references

Gilchrest BA, Eller MS, Geller AC, Yaar M. The pathogenesis of melanoma induced by ultraviolet radiation. *N Engl J Med* 1999; 340:1341–8.

Grossman D, Leffell DJ. The molecular basis of nonmelanoma skin cancer: new understanding. *Arch Dermatol* 1997;133:1263–70.

Tsao H. Genetics of nonmelanoma skin cancer. *Arch Dermatol* 2001; 137:1486–92.

Clinical assessment is fundamental to the diagnostic process. This begins with the patient history. A story of changing, enlarging and irritating lesions should alert suspicion. Patients who present with a skin cancer invariably describe a growth that is changing. It is reassuring to hear that a lesion is longstanding and is not changing.

Rigorous systematic clinical examination is mandatory to elicit key morphologic features (size, shape, symmetry, surface, margin, color, texture) of benign or malignant skin tumors.

A clear diagnosis of a skin tumor is usually attained after clinical assessment, but histology is regarded as the gold standard.

The dermatoscope, or surface microscope, is a handheld instrument that assists with the examination of cutaneous lesions. Generally, this light magnification system has a fixed magnification of × 10. Oil is usually applied to the skin lesion to reduce light refraction; however, newer systems with cross-polarized light enable examination without oil. The instrument was developed to aid the examination of pigmented lesions, but its precise role is under evaluation.

Biopsy and histology

Biopsy and histological examination are integral to the diagnosis of skin cancer.

Shave biopsy. When the skin lesion is pedunculated and only appears to involve the epidermis and upper dermis, a superficial slice of skin can be removed with a scalpel or razor blade. Sutures are not usually required and electrodesiccation or aluminum chloride may be applied to achieve hemostasis. The procedure only leaves a small scab that heals in 2–4 weeks.

Punch biopsy. Dermatologists are enthusiasts for this biopsy, and use it for suspected skin dermatoses, BCC, SCC and actinic keratoses. A circular blade attached to a handle is rotated through the skin, capturing a core of tissue. The core is removed and sent to the laboratory for histological assessment. Once the biopsy has been taken, the residual skin defect can be closed with sutures or steri-strips. Alternatively, the wound can be left to re-epithelialize and heal by secondary intention. A range of skin biopsy diameters is available, but in most situations a punch biopsy diameter of 3–6 mm is appropriate.

Incisional biopsy. For this procedure, an ellipse of tissue is removed using a surgical blade, so that a proportion of the lesion can be sent for histological assessment. The remaining defect is usually repaired with sutures.

Excisional biopsy. The entire lesion is removed. The excision is usually elliptical.

Benign lesions

Acquired melanocytic nevus. This type of nevus usually becomes apparent after the age of 12, increasing in number over the next 20 years, before starting to dissipate. There are several types of acquired nevi:
- junctional
- compound
- intradermal
- halo
- pigmented spindle cell nevus of Reed
- Spitz
- blue.

Junctional nevi usually develop in adolescents, compound nevi in young adults and intradermal nevi in older adults. This observation has led to the hypothesis that throughout life the nevomelanocyte composition progresses from a junctional nevus to a compound nevus and then on to an intradermal nevus.

Junctional nevus. This type of nevus most commonly arises in childhood and early adulthood. It is a flat, sharply demarcated,

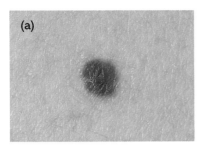

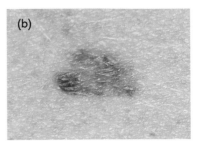

Figure 3.1 Junctional nevus: a flat, pigmented lesion, usually < 6 mm in diameter.

pigmented lesion, usually with a diameter of less than 6 mm (Figure 3.1). Junctional nevi often develop on palms and soles and tend to maintain the normal skin markings. Histologically, discrete nests of nevomelanocytes can be found in contact with the basal layer of the epidermis.

Compound nevus. This is a slightly elevated, well-delineated, pigmented lesion, most commonly found in adults (Figure 3.2). It tends to have a uniform color in the range of tan to dark brown. A proportion of the nevomelanocytes are free within the papillary dermis, whereas others are in contact with the overlying epidermal basal layer.

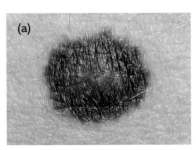

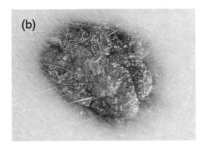

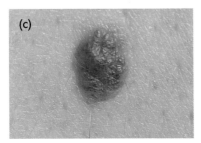

Figure 3.2 Compound nevus: an elevated, well-delineated, pigmented lesion, which tends to have a uniform color, ranging from tan to dark brown.

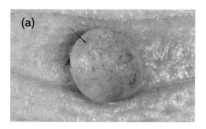

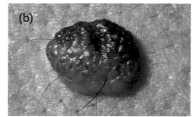

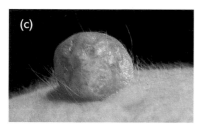

Figure 3.3 Intradermal nevus: a fleshy nodule or skin tag with minimal pigmentation, commonly found on the face.

Intradermal nevus. This tends to be a fleshy nodule or skin tag, with minimal pigmentation, commonly found on the face of older adults (Figure 3.3). Histological examination shows that the nevomelanocyte nests are free within the dermis and there is no involvement of the overlying epidermis.

Halo nevus, also termed Sutton's nevus, has a characteristic ring of hypopigmentation encircling the central pigmented nevus (Figure 3.4). The pigment loss is a consequence of an autoimmune assault on the compound nevus. This nevus, if not excised, will involute spontaneously over a few months; however, the depigmentation may persist for some years. Halo nevi most frequently develop on the trunks of adolescents and young adults.

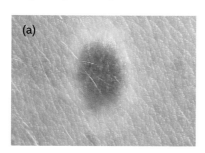

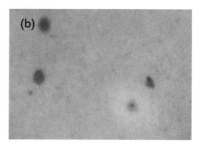

Figure 3.4 Halo nevus: (a) with a ring of hypopigmentation encircling the central pigmented nevus; (b) among multiple nevi on the back.

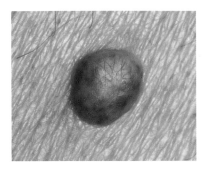

Figure 3.5 Spitz nevus: a rapidly growing, firm, orange-red papule, which commonly presents on the face.

Pigmented spindle cell nevus of Reed is a blue-black, heavily pigmented nevus, seen more commonly in women than men, often on the thigh. Histologically, these lesions are comprised of spindle nevus cells with highly concentrated melanin.

Spitz nevus presents classically as a rapidly growing, firm, orange-red papule on the face. This compound nevus variant develops principally in children and young adults. It can be difficult to differentiate histologically from melanoma, and pathologists must exercise extreme caution if making the diagnosis in older individuals (Figure 3.5).

Blue nevus. This is a small, uniform lesion of an intense black-blue color. It may be a macule, papule or plaque (Figure 3.6). Blue nevi are thought to arise from dermal melanocytes that did not complete their migration from the neural crest to the dermoepidermal junction during embryology.

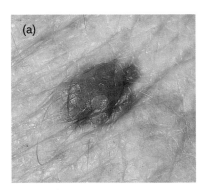
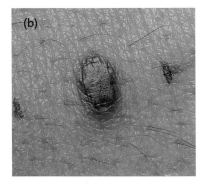

Figure 3.6 Blue nevus: a small, uniform lesion of an intense black-blue color, presenting as a macule, papule or plaque.

Seborrheic keratosis is a benign lesion generally seen in older individuals. It arises from epidermal keratinocytes and is variable in its clinical presentation (Figure 3.7). The lesion is usually elevated, warty and hyperkeratotic, and tends to reach a diameter of 10–30 mm.

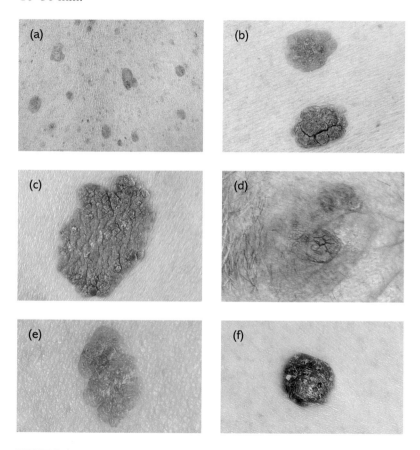

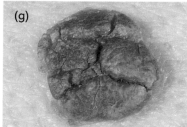

Figure 3.7 Seborrheic keratosis is variable in appearance, and reaches diameters of 10–30 mm: (a) multiple; (b) and (c) verrucous; (d) diffuse facial; (e) lightly pigmented; (f) deeply pigmented; (g) classic 'stuck-on' appearance.

31

Although generally uniform, the color may range from light brown to black. These are not melanocytic lesions: they obtain their pigment from melanosomes transferred to the keratinocytes from melanocytes. Seborrheic keratoses can be differentiated clinically from melanocytic lesions because they have a verrucous surface, contain keratin horns and have an elevated, 'stuck-on' appearance.

Dermatofibroma. This benign dermal tumor presents as a firm papule or nodule, primarily on the limbs (Figure 3.8). The lesion is well demarcated, ranging from a yellowish color to a dark purplish brown. The color is usually uniform, although there may be increased circumferential pigmentation.

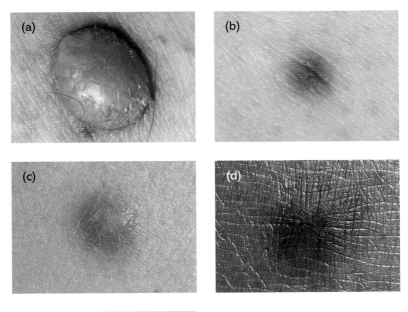

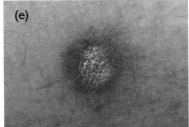

Figure 3.8 Dermatofibroma: a benign dermal tumor that presents as a firm papule or nodule, primarily on the limbs: (a) on ankle; (b) on abdomen; (c) well-demarcated; (d) deeply pigmented; (e) with increased peripheral pigmentation.

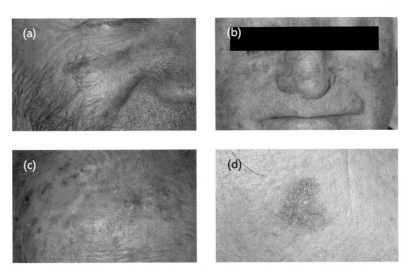

Figure 3.9 Actinic keratosis: a benign scaly patch, papule or plaque that develops on sun-damaged skin: (a) cheek; (b) face; (c) forehead; (d) temple.

Premalignant lesions

Actinic (solar) keratosis is a benign scaly patch, papule or plaque that develops on sun-damaged skin. The lesions may be multiple, and arise predominantly on the face and dorsal aspects of the hands and forearms (Figure 3.9). An individual actinic keratosis characteristically fluctuates in size and can resolve spontaneously. Approximately 5% of lesions progress to SCC over time.

The diagnosis of an actinic keratosis is predominantly clinical. Histology of the lesion is appropriate when the clinical features are not characteristic, and it is important to exclude a cutaneous carcinoma (Figure 3.10). Actinic keratoses present in immunocompromised patients, such as organ transplant recipients

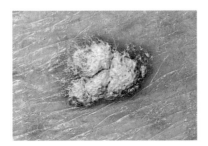

Figure 3.10 Bowenoid actinic keratosis – a small, irregular, keratotic lesion on sun-damaged skin; histology may be necessary to rule out a diagnosis of carcinoma in lesions that lack the characteristic features of an actinic keratosis.

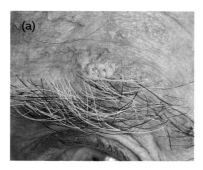
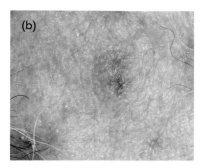

Figure 3.11 Florid actinic keratoses in a patient with chronic lymphocytic leukemia.

and those with human immunodeficiency virus (HIV) infection or chronic lymphocytic leukemia (Figure 3.11). A biopsy is also useful if the actinic keratosis has not responded to standard therapy. The lesions can be easily sampled using a punch biopsy or curette.

Histologically, there is focal parakeratosis, a slight thickening of the epidermis, loss of granular layer and variable alteration in the ordered epidermal architecture.

Keratoacanthoma. This distinctive tumor presents as a rapidly growing, self-resolving hyperkeratotic nodule (Figure 3.12). The lesions usually develop on sun-exposed skin and have three clinical stages:
- proliferation – an initial stage of 2–4 weeks in which the lesion enlarges to more than 20 mm in diameter
- maturation for a few months
- involution – final tumor reabsorption over a further 4–6 months and expulsion of the keratin-filled core.

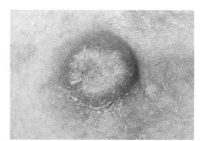

Figure 3.12 Keratoacanthoma on the cheek; this type of lesion is best regarded as a form of SCC and should be treated as such.

(a)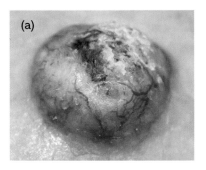

(b)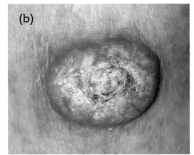

(c)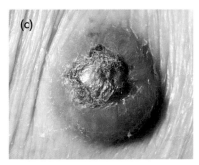

Figure 3.13 Keratoacanthoma has a characteristic, central keratin plug.

Clinically, a keratoacanthoma begins as a smooth papule with slightly erythematous surrounding skin. During the maturation stage, it develops a dome shape with a central keratin plug (Figure 3.13). This plug is later expelled. An atrophic scar often persists after resolution

Although keratoacanthoma is a benign tumor, it can be very difficult to differentiate from SCC, both clinically (Figure 3.14) and histologically. The potential of keratoacanthoma to develop into SCC in the immunosuppressed population is well known.

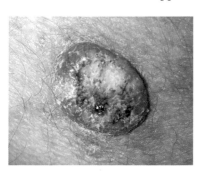

Figure 3.14 A keratoacanthoma-like SCC.

There have also been reports of this phenomenon in non-immunosuppressed individuals. For this reason, keratoacanthomas are usually removed. Removal is achieved by excisional biopsy.

Histological examination of a keratoacanthoma reveals a crater lined with well-differentiated squamous epithelium containing a large central keratin plug. The central keratin component enlarges as the keratoacanthoma matures.

Congenital melanocytic nevus. This type of nevus is present at birth and can be divided into three subgroups depending on its size:

- small congenital nevus, with a widest diameter of less than 15 mm (Figures 3.15 and 3.16)
- medium congenital nevus, with a diameter between 15 and 200 mm (Figure 3.17)
- giant or large nevus, with a widest diameter of more than 200 mm.

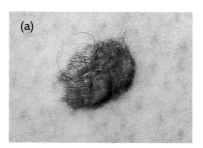
(a)

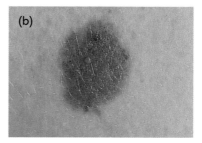
(b)

Figure 3.15 Small congenital melanocytic nevus: widest diameter < 15 mm, with well-demarcated borders. Generally, light brown in infancy, darkening with age.

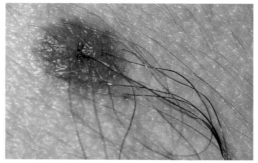

Figure 3.16 A small congenital nevus with a characteristic mammillated surface and terminal hair follicles.

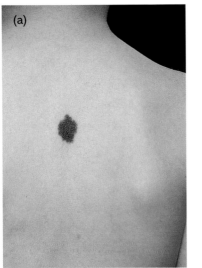
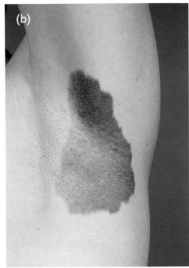

Figure 3.17 Medium congenital melanocytic nevus has a diameter of 15–200 mm.

In infancy, congenital nevi are generally a light-brown color, and they darken with age. These nevi tend to exhibit a mammillated surface and terminal hair follicles (see Figure 3.16), and their borders are usually well demarcated.

Congenital nevi have a greater risk of malignant transformation than acquired nevi. This risk is proportional to the nevus size.

Speckled lentiginous nevus (nevus spilus) may also be present at birth (Figure 3.18). Clinical examination reveals the characteristic hyperpigmented speckles within a light-brown macule, which distinguish this lesion from the congenital melanocytic nevus.

Figure 3.18 Speckled lentiginous nevus (nevus spilus) – characteristic hyperpigmented speckles within a light-brown macule.

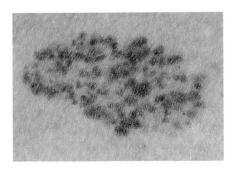

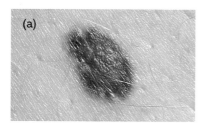

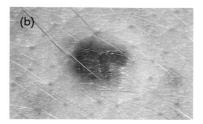

Figure 3.19 Atypical nevi display varied pigmentation and irregular borders.

Atypical nevus syndrome. Clinically, an atypical nevus can resemble a superficial spreading melanoma. Atypical nevi display varied pigmentation and irregular borders, and often have diameters of more than 10 mm (Figure 3.19). The nevi sometimes develop in unusual sites (Figure 3.20), and they often occur as multiple lesions (Figure 3.21), unlike melanomas, which usually present as single lesions. People with atypical nevi have an increased risk of developing melanoma.

Lentigo maligna (Hutchinson's freckle) is a benign pigmented lesion that clinically begins as a small freckle and slowly enlarges. These brown patches have an irregular border and variegated coloration

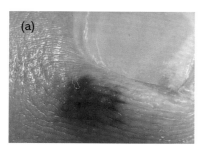

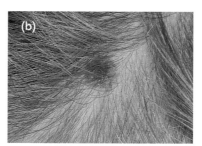

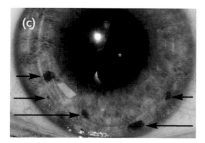

Figure 3.20 Atypical nevi can occur at unusual sites: (a) at the edge of a finger nail; (b) on the scalp; (c) within the iris – iris lentigines (arrowed).

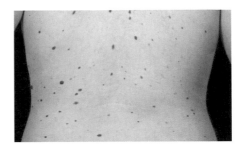

Figure 3.21 Atypical nevus syndrome, with characteristic multiple lesions.

(Figure 3.22). They arise on sun-exposed skin, usually the head or neck, and develop mainly in people over 60 years old. Dark nodules or new, indurated, pigmented papules may arise after a time, a sign of malignant transformation. Approximately 5% of these lesions progress to lentigo maligna melanoma, a tumor with metastatic potential (see page 52).

A biopsy is essential to diagnose lentigo maligna, as the differential diagnosis includes benign pigmented patches such as solar and senile lentigines (Figure 3.23). Like all suspect pigmented lesions, these are best sampled by an excisional biopsy with a narrow margin. If the lesion is too large for an excisional biopsy, an incisional biopsy may be appropriate. However, the portion of the

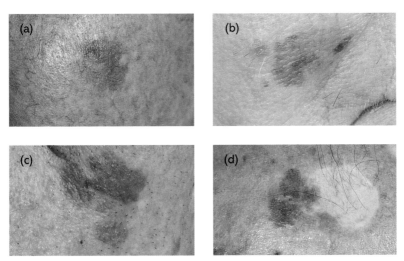

Figure 3.22 Lentigo maligna: a brown patch with variegated color and irregular borders: (a)–(c) on the face; (d) a recurrent lentigo maligna on the scalp.

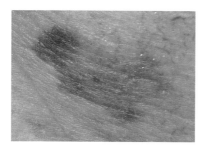

Figure 3.23 A senile lentigo, which has blander, more even pigmentation than lentigo maligna.

tumor sampled with an incisional biopsy may not be representative of the entire lesion. The histology of lentigo maligna is discussed in the section on lentigo maligna melanoma (see page 52).

Xeroderma pigmentosum is one of a number of conditions resulting from abnormal DNA repair. In affected individuals, the risk of developing skin cancer is increased a thousandfold.

The initial clinical presentation is exaggerated sunburn within the first 2 years of life. Children then develop pigmented macules, atrophy and scarring on sun-exposed sites. The predominant cutaneous malignancies are BCC and SCC, although the incidence of melanoma is significantly increased in these children.

Malignant lesions

Basal cell carcinoma (BCC) is the most common human malignancy: it accounts for approximately three-quarters of all skin cancers. The majority of BCCs arise on the head and neck (Figure 3.24).

Variants. BCC can be subdivided into a number of clinico-pathological variants:
- nodular (solid)
- micronodular
- superficial
- pigmented
- adenocystic
- morpheic (sclerosing)
- infiltrative
- basosquamous.

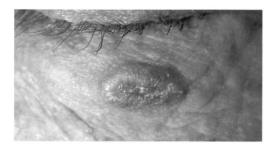

Figure 3.24 BCC usually arises on the head and neck.

Solid or nodular BCC is the most common variant, and develops predominantly on the face (Figure 3.25). A solid BCC initially appears as a translucent, pearly nodule that slowly enlarges. Classically, the lesion is shiny and well-defined, containing dilated superficial capillaries (Figure 3.26). These vessels are located in the thin layer of epithelium that covers the tumor, an area that may periodically scale, erode or crust.

When a BCC diameter is greater than 5 mm, there is a tendency for central ulceration to occur. A large nodular BCC often has a

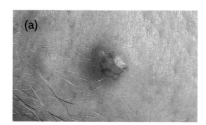

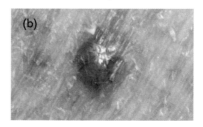

Figure 3.25 Nodular BCC: (a) on the nose, displaying superficial capillaries; (b) on the earlobe.

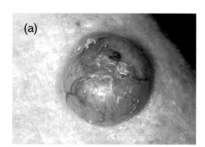

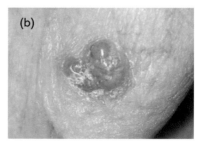

Figure 3.26 Nodular or solid BCC presents as a shiny, well-defined papule or nodule containing dilated superficial capillaries.

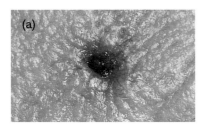
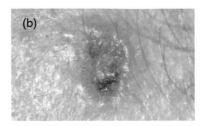

Figure 3.27 Ulcerated BCC: (a) ulceration may occur when the nodule diameter reaches more than 5 mm; (b) large nodule exhibiting a classic rolled, pearly edge.

characteristic pearly rolled appearance at the lesion periphery (Figure 3.27), which can be accentuated by stretching the skin.

Micronodular BCC resembles solid BCC but differs histologically and has a higher risk of recurrence after treatment.

Superficial BCC, which usually arises on the trunk, accounts for 10% of all BCC (Figure 3.28). The lesions extend superficially and are well-defined with a thread-like raised edge. The thin plaques may display central atrophy or scaling, making it difficult to differentiate them from in-situ SCCs. Peripheral islands of tumor and pigmentation are not uncommon.

Pigmented BCC is usually a superficial, micronodular or nodular variant that demonstrates obvious pigmentation (Figure 3.29). It may be brown, red or black, and either completely or irregularly pigmented. The pigmentation is a result of trapped melanin or altered blood composition, and occurs in 2–5% of all BCCs.

Adenocystic BCC tends to present clinically as a diffuse plaque with a rolled edge. Cystic components of this tumor have a more translucent appearance.

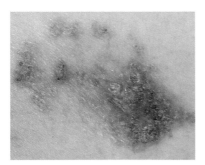

Figure 3.28 A superficial BCC on the back, exhibiting a thread-like raised edge; the thin plaques may display central atrophy or scaling.

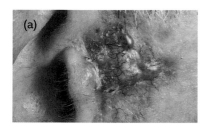

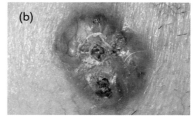

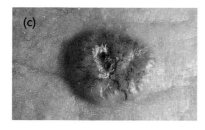

Figure 3.29 Pigmented, nodular BCC; the BCC in (c) is ulcerated.

Morpheic BCC is rare, accounting for only 2% of all BCCs. Occurring almost exclusively on the face, the lesions can be difficult to identify. Morpheic BCC presents as an indurated, scar-like plaque with waxy yellow coloration (Figure 3.30). The margins are ill-defined, and on palpation the BCC is usually considerably larger than it appears on visual inspection (Figure 3.31).

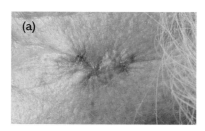

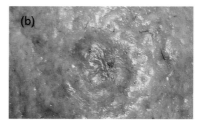

Figure 3.30 Morpheic BCC: (a) displaying scar-like features; (b) presenting as an indurated plaque.

Figure 3.31 A combined solid and morpheic BCC.

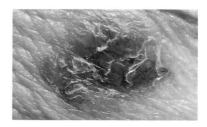

Infiltrative BCC is clinically similar to the morpheic variant in that they both have indistinct borders. However, histologically infiltrative tumor cells are not embedded in the dense fibrous stroma, as occurs in morpheic BCC. Both of these BCC variants are difficult to treat and have higher recurrence rates.

Basosquamous BCC has histological features of both BCC and SCC, but clinically the nodule resembles SCC more than BCC.

Sebaceous nevus complicated by BCC tends to present initially as a nodule within the papillomatous nevus. The risk of developing an associated BCC increases with age, although it has been reported in teenagers.

Nevoid BCC syndrome (Gorlin's syndrome). Patients with Gorlin's syndrome have a mutation – inherited or arising spontaneously in early embryologic development – in one copy of the *patched* (*PTCH*) gene. When the remaining normal copy of the gene is damaged (e.g. by UV or X-ray exposure) a cancer develops.

Classically, patients have multiple BCCs, which are located most commonly on the eyelids, nose, cheeks and forehead, often at symmetrical sites (Figure 3.32). Although these tumors may be present at birth or develop in infancy, they are not usually identified until adolescence.

The BCCs are predominantly nodular and have a benign course similar to sporadic BCC. Other clinical features of Gorlin's

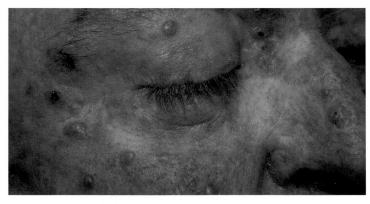

Figure 3.32 Multiple BCCs located on the eyelids and cheeks of a patient with Gorlin's syndrome.

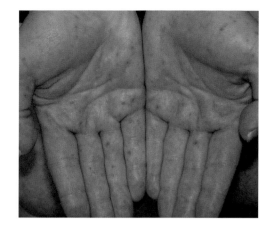

Figure 3.33 Palmoplantar hyperkeratosis and pits in a patient with Gorlin's syndrome.

syndrome include palmoplantar hyperkeratosis and depressions in the skin surface (pits) (Figure 3.33), dental cysts, frontal bossing and abnormalities of the vertebrae and ribs. These associations reflect the important role of the *PTCH* gene in skeletal development as well as in skin maintenance.

Diagnosis. Clinical assessment is often sufficient to make the diagnosis, so treatment can be initiated straight away. However, there are situations in which it is difficult to differentiate a BCC clinically from other lesions such as sebaceous hyperplasia (Figure 3.34), dermatofibroma (see Figure 3.8), SCC and amelanotic melanoma (see Figure 3.50). A biopsy is helpful when there is clinical doubt and before referral for specialist treatment.

Treatments such as radiotherapy, Mohs' surgery, photodynamic therapy and topical therapies generally require a baseline histological diagnosis. A biopsy also provides information on the BCC subtype, which may direct management and assist with prognosis.

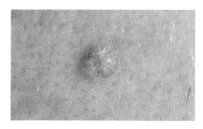

Figure 3.34 Sebaceous hyperplasia – a benign condition in which single or multiple small, yellowish papules develop, usually on the face.

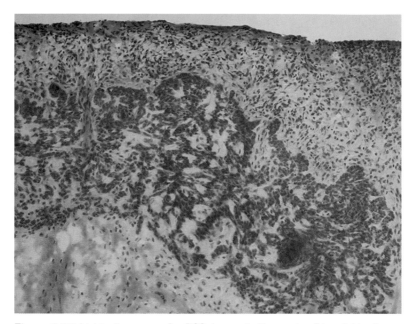

Figure 3.35 Light microscopy of a BCC demonstrating nests of basaloid cells within the dermis.

Histology. The histological features of a BCC vary with the different subtypes. BCC is composed of islands, or nests, of basaloid cells in the dermis, and there is often some attachment to the undersurface of the epidermis (Figure 3.35). The tumor cells have hyperchromatic nuclei with multiple mitoses and sparse cytoplasm. The neoplastic cells in superficial BCC are attached to the epidermis, and are confined to the papillary dermis. In morpheic BCC, the narrow strands of tumor cells are embedded in a dense fibrous stroma.

Metastasis. Most lesions of BCC are small. However, if the presentation is delayed, these tumors can extend from the skin into soft tissue, cartilage and bone. Giant BCC has been known to metastasize on very rare occasions. In these cases, the BCC has usually involved an airway; fragments of tumor have been inhaled, have seeded in the lungs and have developed into metastases. There are a few reports describing cases of hematologic and lymphatic BCC metastases.

Squamous cell carcinoma (SCC) develops on photodamaged skin, usually at sites with the highest exposure to UV radiation. These include the face, neck and dorsum of the hands and forearms. In men, commonly affected sites are the lower lip and pinna, whereas in women the lower legs are frequently involved. SCC can also develop within chronic ulcers or in other situations where cells are constantly stimulated to divide.

In-situ (intraepidermal) SCC. Here, the abnormal keratinocytes are confined to the epidermis. Bowen's disease, first described in 1912, is the most common form of in-situ SCC. Classic Bowen's disease presents as a persistent, slightly scaly, well-demarcated erythematous plaque (Figure 3.36).

The lesions are often isolated and slow growing. Approximately 3% of intraepidermal SCC progress to invasive SCC (Figure 3.37).

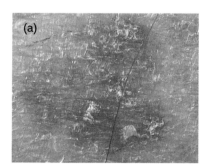 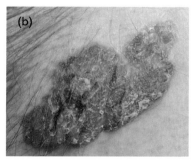

Figure 3.36 Bowen's disease presents as a persistent, slightly scaly, well-demarcated erythematous plaque: (a) on the calf; (b) on the inner thigh.

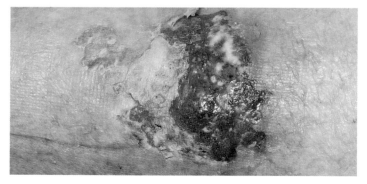

Figure 3.37 Invasive SCC arising in a plaque of Bowen's disease.

47

Other forms of in-situ SCC include those associated with local HPV infection such as bowenoid papulosis and erythroplasia of Queyrat (Figure 3.38). In bowenoid papulosis, men and women develop polymorphic, velvety, warty papules and plaques in the anogenital region. Erythroplasia of Queyrat is a form of penile intraepithelial neoplasia in which red shiny patches or plaques form on the glans penis and prepuce.

Diagnosis. The diagnosis of in-situ SCC is often made clinically. However, a biopsy is helpful in confirming the diagnosis, particularly as many treatments are non-surgical. Tissue sampling with a punch biopsy is adequate and appropriate where there is suspicion of invasive malignancy.

Histology. The histology of in-situ SCC is of atypical keratinocytes throughout the full thickness of the epidermis. The maturation of the epidermis is disorderly, and there is usually an overlying parakeratosis and hyperkeratosis.

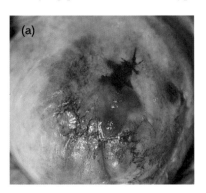

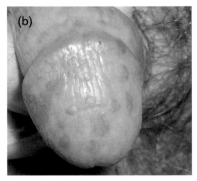

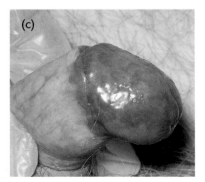

Figure 3.38 (a) Bowen's disease and SCC of the glans penis. A punch biopsy showed high-grade dysplasia, and a deep elliptical biopsy revealed invasive SCC; (b) bowenoid papulosis of the glans penis in a patient with HIV; (c) erythroplasia of Queyrat – SCC in situ of the glans penis.

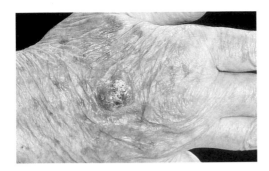

Figure 3.39 Invasive SCC arising in an area of actinic damage on the dorsum of the hand.

Invasive SCC often arises in an area of pre-existing actinic keratosis. The first suspect sign is an ill-defined, firm, indurated lesion (Figure 3.39). This is usually nodular, but it may be plaque-like, verrucous or ulcerated. The tumor is often a yellow-red color with a crusted cap, and will continue to enlarge (Figure 3.40). The surrounding tissue is often inflamed. When mucosal sites are affected, individuals present with non-healing erosions, ulcers or fissures that may bleed intermittently.

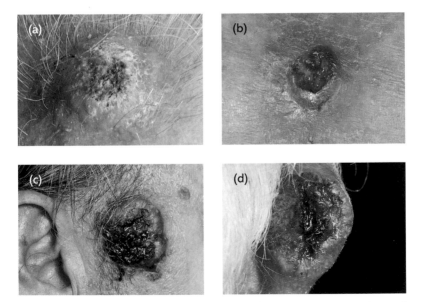

Figure 3.40 Invasive SCC: (a) a recurrent SCC on the forehead; (b) an ulcerated SCC with surrounding inflammation; (c) a large, crusted and ulcerated SCC on the temple; (d) a poorly differentiated SCC on the ear.

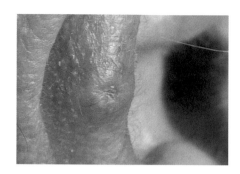

Figure 3.41 Chondrodermatitis nodularis helicis – a painful, benign nodule on the helix of the ear.

Verrucous carcinoma (Buschke–Löwenstein tumor) is a rare, low-grade, well-differentiated SCC. These tumors are warty, vegetating and slow growing. They are typically found in the anogenital region or on the plantar aspect of the foot, although they may also develop in the oral cavity. They rarely metastasize. Invasive SCC can develop in chronic scars, sinuses or ulcers.

Other precursors for invasive SCC include:

- actinic keratosis
- in-situ SCC
- chondrodermatitis nodularis helicis – a small, benign but painful papule on the helix of the ear (Figure 3.41)
- cutaneous horns
- erythema ab igne – a red-brown hyperpigmentation of the skin caused by chronic local exposure to heat.

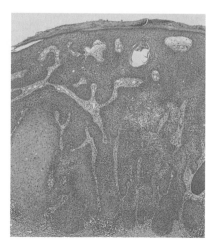

Figure 3.42 Light microscopy of a moderately differentiated, invasive SCC in which dermal nests of atypical squamous epithelial cells arise from the epidermis.

Tumors arising in scars, chronic inflammation or areas of Bowen's disease have an increased risk of metastasizing. Although not as high, there is also an elevated metastatic risk in SCC developing on the lip, ear and non-sun-exposed sites.

Diagnosis. In invasive SCC, the diagnosis is suspected clinically and established histologically. A punch, incisional or, preferably, excisional biopsy can be used.

Histology. Histological examination of an invasive SCC reveals dermal nests of squamous epithelial cells arising from the epidermis (Figure 3.42). There may be associated formations of keratin. The atypical squamous cells have large nuclei with abundant eosinophilic cytoplasm.

The histology report should include the histopathological pattern of SCC, the degree of differentiation with Broders' histological grade, the level of dermal invasion and the presence of perineural, vascular or lymphatic invasion. Information on the margins of the excised tumor is also necessary.

Melanoma. The melanoma subtypes, the incidences of which are shown in Figure 3.43, have distinct clinical presentations. However, the history of an enlarging and changing pigmented lesion is characteristic of most melanomas. Sun exposure is implicated in at least two-thirds of these malignancies.

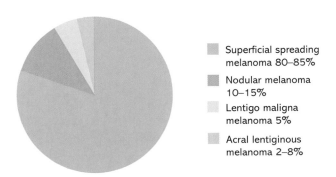

Superficial spreading melanoma 80–85%

Nodular melanoma 10–15%

Lentigo maligna melanoma 5%

Acral lentiginous melanoma 2–8%

Figure 3.43 Relative incidence of the melanoma subtypes.

Lentigo maligna melanoma is found predominantly in older individuals on sun-exposed areas. Around 90% of lesions occur on the head or neck. They develop from the preinvasive lentigo maligna (Hutchinson's melanotic freckle) (see pages 38–40). After a variable period of time, the invasive phase develops within the lentigo maligna, and when the neoplastic melanocytes have extended to the dermis it transforms into a lentigo maligna melanoma (Figure 3.44). At this stage, the neoplasm has metastatic potential. Lentigo maligna melanoma can often be detected clinically as a densely pigmented nodule within the original macular lesion. These nodules can grow rapidly.

Superficial spreading melanoma accounts for approximately 80% of all melanoma. It is observed most frequently on the calves of women and the backs of men.

A typical superficial spreading melanoma is asymmetrical and irregularly outlined. It can be crusted, and presents in different shades of brown, black, red, blue or white (Figure 3.45). The tumor can expand both radially through the epidermis and vertically into the dermis over a period of months or years.

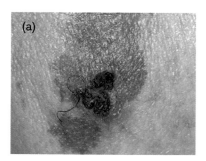

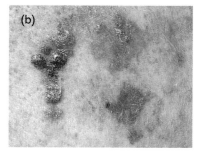

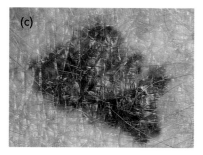

Figure 3.44 Lentigo maligna melanoma: (a) with surrounding lentigo maligna; (b) on a sun-exposed area; (c) complicating the inferior aspect of the lentigo maligna.

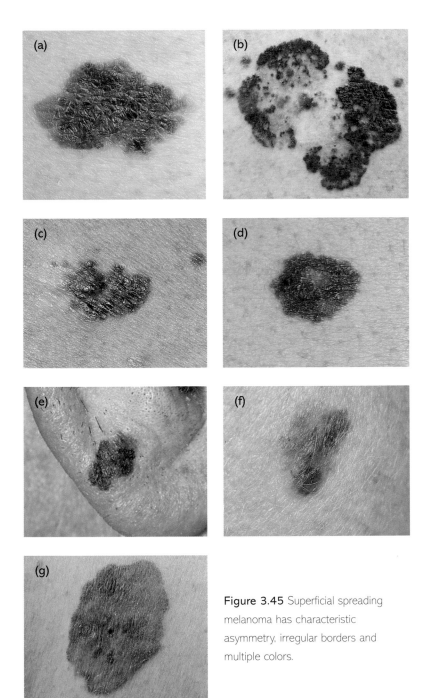

Figure 3.45 Superficial spreading melanoma has characteristic asymmetry, irregular borders and multiple colors.

Nodular melanoma most frequently arises on the trunk and is first observed as a raised black or blue nodular growth (Figure 3.46). Such growths expand rapidly, and the overlying epidermis may ulcerate; it can be difficult to differentiate nodular melanomas from vascular tumors (Figure 3.47).

Acral lentiginous melanoma predominantly occurs in black populations and in people from south east Asia and the Indian subcontinent. Plantar melanoma is more common on the soles than on the palms. It begins as a macule that enlarges and develops a black elevated nodular component. Subungual malignant

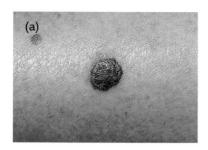

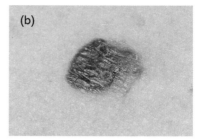

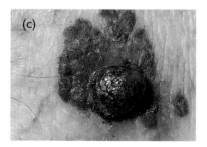

Figure 3.46 Nodular melanoma: (a) with characteristic blue-black pigmentation; (b) developed within a dysplastic nevus, with Breslow thickness 1.2 mm; (c) a combined nodular and superficial spreading melanoma.

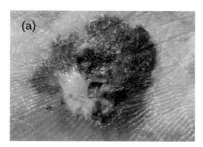

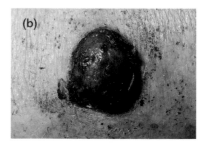

Figure 3.47 Nodular melanoma: (a) displaying crusting and ulceration; (b) with an amelanotic component – may be difficult to differentiate from a vascular tumor.

Figure 3.48 A subungual malignant melanoma exhibiting black pigmentation beneath the nail.

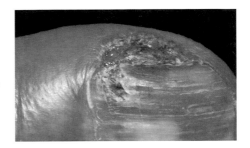

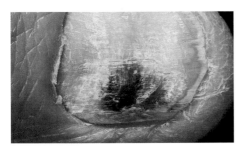

Figure 3.49 A subungual hematoma arising secondary to trauma – not to be confused with a subungual malignant melanoma (see above).

melanoma, with black pigmentation beneath the nail plate, is another form of acral lentiginous melanoma (Figure 3.48). The differential diagnosis includes hemorrhage (Figure 3.49) and fungal infection. Pigmentation of the nail fold is highly suggestive of melanoma and is termed Hutchinson's sign.

Amelanotic melanoma is difficult to identify and should be included in the differential diagnosis of any rapidly growing nodule. Although the name suggests an absence of pigment, amelanotic melanoma usually does have some brown pigmentation to alert the physician to the correct diagnosis (Figure 3.50). They tend to display telangiectasia, and are usually more vascular than intradermal nevi.

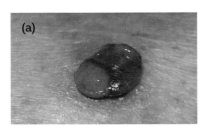

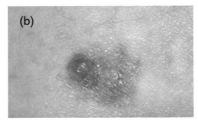

Figure 3.50 (a) An amelanotic melanoma; (b) an amelanotic melanoma with a pigmented component, which can aid diagnosis.

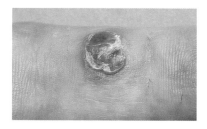

Figure 3.51 Pyogenic granuloma.

Figure 3.52 Cutaneous metastases arising from an internal malignancy.

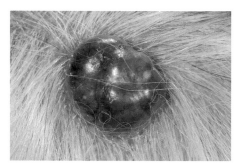

Diagnosis. Early diagnosis of melanoma is essential, as the survival rate decreases with increasing tumor thickness. Clinical diagnosis of malignant melanoma can be difficult, as the differential diagnosis is wide, and includes nevi, seborrheic keratosis, dermato-fibroma, pyogenic granuloma (Figure 3.51), vascular lesions and cutaneous metastases (Figure 3.52). The ABCDEF rule (Table 3.1) is a simple guide that can assist with identifying early melanomas. However, the rule is only a guide, and it should not be applied

TABLE 3.1

Clinical features of melanoma – the ABCDEF rule

A	Lesion asymmetry
B	Irregular border
C	Multiple colors
D	Diameter > 7 mm
E	Evolution/elevation
F	'Funny' mole

TABLE 3.2

Seven-point checklist for melanoma. Melanoma should be suspected if there is any one major feature or any combination of three minor features

Major features	Minor features
Change in size	Diameter ≥ 7 mm
Irregular shape	Inflammation
Irregular color	Oozing
	Change in sensation

strictly – for example, early melanoma may be smaller than 7 mm and there may be no pigment in an amelanotic melanoma.

The UK guidelines for managing cutaneous melanoma promote the use of the seven-point checklist to assist with clinical diagnosis (Table 3.2). This system emphasizes the importance of irregular color or shape and change in size in the identification of suspect lesions.

Dermoscopy. The dermatoscope can assist with the clinical diagnosis of melanoma, enabling examination of the anatomic structures of the epidermis, dermoepidermal junction and superficial papillary dermis. Several pigment patterns that can be seen with this instrument are suggestive of melanoma. The usual approach is to put the dermatoscopic findings into an algorithm to calculate the likelihood of a malignant melanoma. The most commonly used algorithms are the ABCD rule of dermoscopy, the seven-point checklist and Menzies' scoring method (Table 3.3). These have been developed from the initial technique of pattern analysis, and all are recognized as valid methods for evaluating pigmented lesions with dermoscopy. A meta-analysis of the usefulness of dermoscopy for the diagnosis of melanoma concluded that, for formally trained, experienced operators, dermoscopy gave a more accurate diagnosis than clinical examination alone. Although dermoscopy may improve diagnostic accuracy, it has not yet been shown to alter the physician's practice or increase the sensitivity of excision biopsy in malignant melanoma.

TABLE 3.3

Menzies' scoring method for the dermatoscopic diagnosis of invasive melanoma

Melanoma is suspected in a lesion that does not have both reassuring features and has one or more 'worrying' feature:

Reassuring features *(Absent in all melanomas)**	**Symmetry of pattern** through the lesion's radial and longitudinal axes
	Presence of a single color – black, gray, blue, dark brown, tan and red are scored, but white is not scored as a color
Worrying features *(Specificity of > 85% for invasive melanoma)**	**Blue-white veil** – an irregular, structureless area of confluent blue pigmentation with an overlying white 'ground-glass' haze
	Multiple brown dots – focal areas of well-defined dark-brown dots (not globules)
	Pseudopods – bulbous and often kinked projections found at the edge of a lesion directly connected to either the tumor body or pigmented network
	Radial streaming – asymmetrically arranged finger-like extensions at the edge of the lesion
	Scar-like depigmentation – areas of white, discrete, irregular extensions, not to be confused with hypo- or depigmentation caused by simple loss of melanin
	Peripheral black dots/globules – found at or near the edge of the lesion
	Multiple (5–6) colors – black, gray, blue, dark brown, tan and red are scored, but white is not scored as a color
	Multiple blue/gray dots – a 'pepper-like' pattern of blue or gray dots (not globules)
	Broadened network – pigmented network with irregular, thick 'cords', often seem focally thicker

*In Menzies' original training set (Menzies S et al. *Melanoma Res* 1996;6:55–62).
Adapted from Menzies et al. *Arch Dermatol* 1996;132:1178–82.

Biopsy. If there is suspicion of melanoma, a full-thickness excisional biopsy of the tumor should be performed. The UK and US melanoma guidelines recommend that the pigmented lesion under investigation should be excised initially with a narrow margin (2–5 mm) to the depth of subcutaneous fat. Punch and shave biopsies should not be used, as they interfere with histological staging. An incisional biopsy is occasionally appropriate in large lesions on the face suggestive of lentigo maligna or when sampling for subungual melanoma. Incisional biopsy has not been shown to have an adverse effect on survival.

Histopathology. Histopathological assessment is fundamental to the diagnosis of melanoma and should be performed by a pathologist who is experienced in diagnosing pigmented lesions. The histology also provides information on prognosis and directs the therapeutic intervention. The most important prognostic factor is the Breslow thickness of a tumor; it is measured histologically from the top of the granular layer to the deepest tumor cell. Information that should appear in the histopathology report is shown in Table 3.4.

The histopathological features of melanoma differ between subtypes. However, in general, the radial growth phase – the process by which a pigmented lesion extends horizontally – correlates with the proliferation of atypical melanocytes within the epidermis or papillary dermis. This is followed by the vertical growth phase, except in nodular melanoma in which there is no radial growth phase.

Lentigo maligna. The atypical melanocytes are usually confined to the basal layer of the epidermis where they reside singly or in nests and may extend to the adnexal epithelium. This transforms to lentigo maligna melanoma when it develops an invasive component.

Superficial spreading melanoma is characterized by proliferating atypical melanocytes present at all levels of the epidermis.

Nodular melanoma is comprised of a dermal mass of melanoma cells and, although there may be some invasion to the overlying epidermis, the tumor does not have an intraepithelial component.

Physical examination. An individual recently diagnosed with melanoma requires a thorough physical examination to search for any lymphadenopathy, hepatomegaly or other suspect pigmented lesions. If any such abnormalities are identified on physical examination, further investigation is required. There is strong evidence that routine imaging and blood tests have little, if any, value for the asymptomatic patient who has a normal physical examination and a Breslow thickness of 4 mm or less.

Staging. The American Joint Committee on Cancer provides a melanoma staging system that is widely accepted around the world (Table 3.5).

The British melanoma guidelines suggest that no further investigations are required for stage I and stage IIA disease. However, for those with stage IIB or higher they recommend blood tests to check the complete blood count, liver function and lactate dehydrogenase level. For these groups, they also suggest a chest radiograph, liver ultrasound and optional computed tomography scan of the chest and abdomen with or without the pelvis.

TABLE 3.4

Information that should be included in the melanoma histopathology report

- Tumor site
- Surgical procedure undertaken
- Macroscopic examination and dimensions
- Breslow thickness
- Evidence of ulceration
- Degree of radial and/or vertical growth
- Melanoma subtype
- Degree of tumor regression
- Presence of microsatellites
- Statement on completeness of excision with margins

TABLE 3.5

American Joint Committee on Cancer staging system for melanoma

Stage	Primary tumor (Breslow thickness)	Lymph node	Metastases
O	In-situ tumors	Nil	Nil
IA	≤ 1.0 mm, no ulceration	Nil	Nil
IB	≤ 1.0 mm + ulceration	Nil	Nil
	1.01–2.0 mm, no ulceration	Nil	Nil
IIA	1.01–2.0 mm + ulceration	Nil	Nil
	2.01–4.0 mm, no ulceration	Nil	Nil
IIB	2.01–4.0 mm + ulceration	Nil	Nil
	> 4.0 mm, no ulceration	Nil	Nil
IIC	> 4.0 mm + ulceration	Nil	Nil
IIIA	Any thickness, no ulceration	Nodal micrometastases	Nil
IIIB	Any thickness + ulceration	Nodal micrometastases	Nil
	Any thickness, no ulceration	≤ 3 palpable nodes	Nil
	Any thickness ± ulceration	No nodes but in-transit metastases or satellites	Nil
IIIC	Any thickness + ulceration	≤ 3 palpable nodes	Nil
	Any thickness ± ulceration	≥ 4 palpable nodes, matted nodes or nodes and in-transit metastases	Nil
IV:M1		Distant nodes	Skin or sub-cutaneous metastases
IV:M2			Lung metastases
IV:M3			Other sites or metastases at any site and raised lactate dehydrogenase

Adapted from Balch et al. 2003.

Treatments

Most tumors are surgically excised. However, there are a number of different treatments that may be suitable for patients with premalignant or malignant cutaneous lesions. These include:

- topical preparations
- cryotherapy
- curettage and electrosurgery
- Mohs' micrographic surgery
- photodynamic therapy (PDT) and lasers
- radiotherapy.

Topical therapies may be sufficient to treat premalignant and malignant cutaneous lesions.

Topical 5-fluorouracil cream is an established treatment for actinic keratosis, superficial BCC and in-situ SCC. The mode of action is thought to be a direct cytotoxic effect on neoplastic cells.

Topical 3% diclofenac sodium gel is a non-steroidal anti-inflammatory agent that is licensed in the USA and UK for the treatment of actinic keratosis. Although experience with this product is limited, it appears to be of value.

Topical imiquimod cream is a novel immunomodulatory agent licensed in the UK for the treatment of small superficial BCC. Imiquimod and other imidazoquinolones activate antigen-presenting cells, inducing secretion of proinflammatory cytokines. Interferon α, tumor necrosis factor α and interleukin-12 have a central role in mediating the resultant cytotoxic effect. Studies have demonstrated the antitumor effects of imiquimod when it is applied to cutaneous lesions.

Cryotherapy is an easily administered treatment for a number of cutaneous premalignant and malignant lesions. Of the cryogens, liquid nitrogen (which boils at −196°C) is the most effective for treating skin cancer; when it is used clinically, intra- and extracellular ice crystals form, causing cell rupture and tissue destruction. The liquid nitrogen is contained in a handheld unit and is applied to the skin via a spray or probe. It is best directed at areas with a diameter of 6 mm or less – small lesions or discrete areas within larger lesions. In this way, the epidermis and dermis are frozen effectively.

There is variation in technique between cryosurgeons: some prefer a continuous-freeze technique, whereas others apply the spray in pulses. The period in seconds during which the liquid nitrogen is applied and the number of freeze–thaw cycles depends on the lesion. After cryotherapy a moist wound usually develops, which may become ulcerated, and there is subsequent crusting and scab formation. After the wound has healed completely, an area of altered pigmentation or frank scarring may remain.

Curettage and electrosurgery. A curette has an oval or cup-shaped component with a cutting edge and a handle. The original curette was developed in the late 1800s; over the years it has proved an invaluable tool for the dermatologist. When combined with electrosurgery, the curette is an effective treatment for many non-melanoma skin cancers.

There are two types of electrosurgical technique:
- electrodesiccation
- electrocautery.

In electrodesiccation, a monoterminal provides a high voltage and low amperage, both of which are superficially destructive to the skin. This technique differs from electrocautery in which a biterminal supplies a low voltage and high amperage, producing a more deeply destructive effect on the skin.

Although there have been no studies comparing the two, curettage is usually combined with electrodesiccation rather than electrocautery. Because electrodesiccation is only superficially destructive, in combination with curettage it is considered to result in reduced scarring and improved cosmesis, and to make treatment of recurrences easier.

Although there is some variation in the technique of curettage and electrosurgery, the general principles are consistent.

Curettage. After the initial injection of local anesthetic, the tumor is debulked with a medium- or large-sized curette. This is repeatedly drawn through the tumor, including its base. A smaller curette is then used for the margins to ensure the removal of the maximal number of tumor cells. After the neoplasm has been removed, there is a change in tissue consistency – the coarse resistance of normal tissue can be distinguished.

Saucerization curettage refers to removal of the tumor in one pass to create a deep saucer-shaped wound.

Electrodesiccation is applied to the base and to an extra 2 mm beyond the rim after satisfactory curettage. This procedure is then repeated. Two or three passes of curettage and electrodesiccation are thought to be adequate for treating non-melanoma skin cancer. One, more superficial, pass suffices for an actinic keratosis.

Outcome. The resulting wounds heal by secondary intention over a 6-week period. Potential side effects include atrophic or hypertrophic scarring, tissue contraction and altered pigmentation at the scar site. Overall, though, this is a safe and effective treatment for many non-melanoma cutaneous malignancies.

Micrographic surgery was developed in the 1940s by Frederick Mohs. The technique relies on the fundamental principle that when a tumor is removed with histological margin control, maximal confidence in the completeness of the excision can be combined with minimal loss of surrounding normal tissue. Mohs' original procedure involved removing the tumor, fixing the tissue and then sectioning the excision margins to reach any tumor involvement. He had excellent cure rates. Today, his technique has been modified: tissue is generally frozen immediately and sectioned, curtailing the length of the procedure (Figure 4.1).

The excised tissue sections and the surgical sites are carefully labeled and oriented so that, following histological examination, the potential locations of residual tumor can be identified. Further sections are then taken according to the histological findings, and

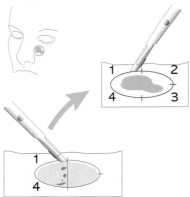

Stage 1: The tumor is debulked and a thin layer of skin is excised from the surrounding skin and base.

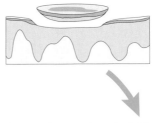

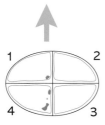

Stages 1 to 4 are repeated where residual tumor remains (surrounding normal tissue is spared) until the skin is clear of tumor. When the tumor is completely removed, the skin defect is repaired.

Stage 2: The specimen is divided into tissue slices, which are numbered or color-coded on a 'Mohs' map' relating the specimen's orientation to the surgical defect; the tissue slices are then frozen.

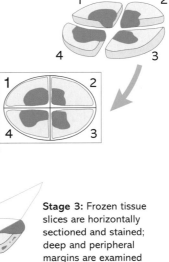

Stage 4: From the map, residual tumor is located on the wound, marked and removed.

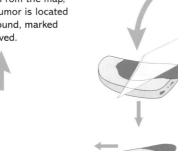

Stage 3: Frozen tissue slices are horizontally sectioned and stained; deep and peripheral margins are examined under the microscope to determine if the whole tumor has been removed. Any evidence of tumor is located on the map.

Figure 4.1 The stages of Mohs' micrographic surgery.

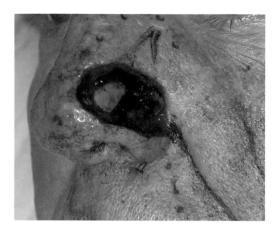

Figure 4.2 Mohs' micrographic surgery, in which the tumor has been completely excised and reconstruction can begin.

the process is repeated until the surgeon is satisfied that the lesion has been excised completely. At this point, surgical repair of the wound can commence (Figure 4.2). Mohs' micrographic surgery is usually performed under local anesthesia and completed within 5 hours.

The procedure is generally reserved for recurrent tumors and those with an infiltrative growth pattern located at critical anatomic sites.

Photodynamic therapy (PDT) has proved to be an effective treatment for some non-melanoma skin cancers. A histological diagnosis is usually obtained first. The technique involves activating a tissue-localized photosensitizer by visible light, resulting in cell damage and death. The optimal topical agent and disease-specific irradiance are yet to be established.

Experience in cutaneous PDT has been gained using topical 5-aminolevulinic acid (5-ALA), which is licensed in the USA for the treatment of actinic keratosis. 5-ALA is applied to lesions for 1–18 hours, with or without occlusion. It appears to be taken up selectively by and/or retained in diseased tissue during this period and converted to the photosensitizer protoporphyrin IX. The lesion is then illuminated with a laser or incoherent light source within the visible spectrum, with wavelengths in the Soret band (400–410 nm, blue light) being the most effective in triggering the photodynamic reaction.

A number of derivatives of 5-ALA have been synthesized to develop compounds that penetrate the plasma membrane of the target cells and diffuse through epidermal layers more easily. Methyl aminolevulinate (MAL), an ester of ALA, is more lipophilic than free ALA and penetrates more effectively through cutaneous tissue. In an optimal regimen, MAL, 160 mg/g, is applied for 3 hours under an occlusive dressing before illumination with red light (570–670 nm). It is licensed in Europe and Australia for the treatment of actinic keratosis and BCC (both nodular and superficial), and in the USA for non-hyperkeratotic actinic keratosis.

PDT can be painful and produces a dose-dependent phototoxicity reaction (erythema and edema) that lasts several days. Otherwise, PDT has relatively few side effects, and the final cosmesis appears to be good.

Lasers can be used for destruction of precancerous lesions and established non-melanoma skin cancer.

Radiotherapy is a well-established treatment for cutaneous malignances. Skin cancer is generally treated with conventional radiotherapy using X-rays, which are more penetrating and have a shorter wavelength than both visible and UV radiation.

Suspect lesions are biopsied and a histological diagnosis is confirmed before radiotherapy. The degree to which radiotherapy is employed for skin-cancer therapy varies between centers.

Radiosensitive neoplasms include BCC, SCC and some vascular tumors. Radiotherapy is not as effective for melanoma, but its role in lentigo maligna is under reappraisal. Radiotherapy is particularly useful for large neoplasms and those located on the ears, nose and lower eyelid. It is best avoided on the lower legs, at sites subject to repeated trauma and on skin overlying susceptible organs such as the thyroid.

Radiotherapy is a valuable option for the frail elderly, but in younger patients the long-term side effects of skin atrophy, scarring and telangiectasia can make the results cosmetically inferior to those achieved with surgery. In addition, because X-rays are themselves carcinogenic, there is a risk of eventual therapy-induced cancer. Finally, previous radiotherapy makes subsequent surgery more challenging.

Management of at-risk patients

It is important to identify those individuals who are at high risk of cutaneous malignancies so that management strategies for them can be implemented. Management strategies are needed for patients with:

- benign lesions that may become malignant
- premalignant lesions
- substantial previous UV radiation exposure/chronic photodamage
- immunosuppression
- a genetic predisposition for cutaneous malignancies.

Benign lesions

Congenital melanocytic nevus. This type of nevus has a higher potential for malignant transformation than an acquired nevus. The lifetime risk of melanoma is not well established, but for small to medium-sized congenital nevi (see Figures 3.15–3.17) it is thought to be 0–5%, with melanoma usually developing at, or after, puberty. For large congenital nevi the lifetime risk is 5–12%, and the melanoma usually arises before puberty.

The management of congenital melanocytic nevi is not well defined and should be individualized. Excision of giant nevi is often not feasible, but where it is, it should take place early in life. In contrast, the prophylactic excision of medium and small congenital nevi can be planned for any age up to puberty, although it is not usual practice to excise all small congenital nevi.

If medium-sized or giant nevi are not removed, self-examination and periodic surveillance, with photographs, are required. Individuals with large congenital nevi or multiple satellite nevi located over the spine, neck or head are at increased risk of

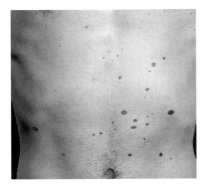 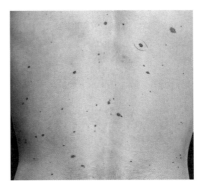

Figure 4.3 Surveillance photographs of a patient with atypical nevus syndrome; these assist the examiner or patient in the identification of changing nevi.

neurocutaneous melanocytosis, with the associated problems of hydrocephalus or seizures. These deposits can be identified with magnetic resonance imaging.

Atypical nevus syndrome. The presence of atypical nevi is a significant risk factor for melanoma (see Figures 3.19–3.21). The risk is lower in a patient with only one or two atypical moles and no family history of melanoma than in a patient who has both atypical nevi and a family history of atypical nevi and melanoma (familial atypical mole and melanoma syndrome). The term 'atypical nevus syndrome' is used to represent this spectrum of phenotypic expression.

Individuals with atypical nevi should be encouraged to perform self-examinations every 1–3 months to look for changes in their moles. Surveillance of their nevi by a doctor is also recommended and can be aided by cutaneous photographs (Figure 4.3). The importance of protection from the sun must be emphasized and family members should also be screened.

Spitz nevus. The optimal management of a Spitz nevus is not clearly defined. Although the nevus is benign (see Figure 3.5), it can be difficult to exclude melanoma definitively. For this reason, an excisional biopsy with re-excision of any positive margins is probably the treatment of choice.

Genetic predisposition and other 'at-risk' factors

Genetic counseling should be offered to individuals with nevoid BCC syndrome, xeroderma pigmentosum and the xeroderma pigmentosum variants.

Xeroderma pigmentosum. Patients with xeroderma pigmentosum are managed with strict photoprotection including sun avoidance, a daily sunscreen, self-examination and regular surveillance by their dermatologist. Oral retinoids such as isotretinoin or acitretin have a prophylactic role. A topical preparation of a DNA-repair enzyme is under evaluation.

Nevoid BCC syndrome (Gorlin's syndrome). Individuals with Gorlin's syndrome require vigilant dermatological surveillance (see Figures 3.32–3.33). Early diagnosis is advantageous, as strict photo-protective measures can then be instituted from a young age. However, as a high rate of disease arises from spontaneous mutations, early diagnosis can be difficult. Treatment of BCC is similar to that for BCC in an unaffected individual, except that radiotherapy is avoided.

Immunosuppression. Cutaneous malignancies associated with iatrogenic immunosuppression and HIV infection can be atypical and aggressive (Figure 4.4a). A high index of suspicion is required when examining immunocompromised patients, with a low threshold for skin biopsies. In addition, this population requires regular skin surveillance and education about strict sun protection.

Substantial UV radiation exposure. Individuals who have received a large cumulative dose of UV radiation or episodic UV radiation burns are at increased risk of skin cancer. If there is a history of severe sunburn, significant sun exposure or sunbed use (Figure 4.4b), particularly in lighter skin types that are sensitive to sunlight (types I and II), the patient should be offered education on sun protection and self-examination.

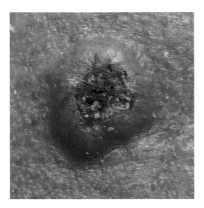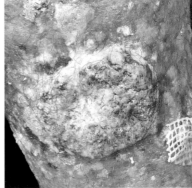

Figure 4.4 SCC: (a) in an organ transplant recipient; (b) associated with excessive sunbed use.

Premalignant lesions

Actinic keratosis. Treatment options include:

- cryotherapy
- topical diclofenac
- topical 5-fluorouracil
- topical 5% imiquimod
- PDT.

Cryotherapy. Actinic keratoses (see Figures 3.9–3.11) are usually treated with cryotherapy. Normally, actinic keratoses respond to a single freeze–thaw cycle with a freezing time of 5–15 seconds. Although this is an excellent therapy, there is associated discomfort and a permanent hypopigmented patch can develop after treatment.

Topical 3% diclofenac sodium is a gel with efficacy in the treatment of actinic keratoses. It is applied to the lesion twice daily for 60 to 90 days. Although generally well tolerated, this preparation is contraindicated in those with an allergy to non-steroidal anti-inflammatory agents.

Topical 5-fluorouracil is an effective therapy for actinic keratoses, although it can cause erythema and discomfort over several weeks.

Topical 5% imiquimod has been shown, in recent studies, to be a useful agent. It is a treatment option in the USA for certain patients with actinic keratosis.

Photodynamic therapy (PDT) also has proven value. MAL PDT has shown efficacy in all locations and grades of actinic keratosis, whereas 5-ALA PDT is best directed at non-hyperkeratotic actinic keratoses on the face.

Curettage and/or electrocautery is used by many dermatologists.

Keratoacanthoma (see Figures 3.12–3.13). Treatment options include:
- surgical excision
- curettage and electrosurgery
- Mohs' micrographic surgery.

As it is difficult to differentiate keratoacanthoma from invasive SCC (see Figure 3.14), both clinically and histologically, it is prudent to employ SCC treatments for these lesions (see pages 77–80). Keratoacanthoma is therefore most commonly excised surgically, but curettage and electrosurgery may be appropriate for small, classic lesions.

Keratoacanthoma developing on the central face is characteristically more aggressive and Mohs' micrographic surgery warrants consideration.

Lentigo maligna. If left untreated, a small proportion of cases of lentigo maligna (see Figures 3.22–3.23) will progress to lentigo maligna melanoma (see Figure 3.44).

Treatment options include:
- conventional surgical excision
- Mohs' micrographic surgery
- cryotherapy
- topical imiquimod.

The mainstay of treatment is conventional surgical excision with a 5–10 mm surgical margin, although the highest cure rates are seen using Mohs' micrographic surgery. Cryotherapy has been used, and recent reports describe success with topical imiquimod. The place of radiotherapy has been the subject of re-evaluation recently. In elderly patients, particularly those with a large facial lesion, observation of the lentigo maligna may be the most appropriate approach.

Malignant lesions

Basal cell carcinoma. There are a number of effective treatments available for BCC, both surgical and non-surgical, which are discussed below. Factors such as the patient's preference, age and health, as well as the clinical and histological subtype, size and site need to be considered when making a management decision (see Figures 3.24–3.31). The non-surgical treatments (radiotherapy, topical 5-fluorouracil, topical imiquimod and PDT) have the disadvantage of not generating a pathological specimen. Therefore, a histological diagnosis cannot be ascertained for patients treated by non-surgical means.

Surgical excision is the most common treatment for primary BCC and is very effective. It is the treatment of choice for most recurrent, nodular, morpheic or superficial facial BCCs, but indications for Mohs' micrographic surgery should be absent. It is useful to curette the BCC before excision so that the 'naked eye' tumor margin can be delineated.

The optimal excision margin depends on the BCC subtype and size. For a primary BCC with a diameter of less than 2 cm, there is evidence that a 3-mm surgical excision margin will clear the tumor in 85% of cases, a rate that increases to 95% clearance with a margin of 4–5 mm. The excision margin must be wider for morpheic and large BCCs. Similar studies show that a morpheic BCC excised with a margin of 5 mm has an 82% peripheral clearance rate; however, with a margin of 13–15 mm, the rate improves to over 95% clearance. Recurrent BCCs also have lower cure rates, and excision margins of 5–10 mm have been suggested.

There is controversy over the management of incompletely excised BCC. The tumor does not necessarily have to be totally removed to achieve complete resolution. Studies have shown wide variation in the risk of recurrence, from 16% to 60%. The risk appears to be lower if the lateral margins are involved rather than the deeper margin.

The general opinion is that observation is sensible for the patient with a non-aggressive subtype of BCC that is incompletely excised on a lateral margin.

Mohs' micrographic surgery is a labor-intensive, specialized procedure (see Figure 4.1) that achieves very high BCC cure rates: 99% 5-year cure rate for primary BCC and 94% for recurrent BCC. This treatment is reserved for aggressive histological BCC subtypes located on critical or high-risk sites. It is not mandated for all BCC because it is time-consuming and expensive, and the morbidity may exceed the benefit. Table 4.1 lists features of a BCC that may indicate consideration of Mohs' micrographic surgery.

Curettage with electrosurgery is a valuable treatment for small, well-defined, primary BCCs that have a non-aggressive histology and are not located on critical sites; the 5-year cure rate for this treatment has been shown to be as high as 97%. The cure rates are variable and seem to be operator dependent. Studies show overall cure rates to be 92% after 5 years for primary BCC and 60% for recurrent BCC. Curettage and electrosurgery may not be successful for recurrent or morpheic BCC.

Cryosurgery is best reserved for the treatment of extrafacial superficial BCC; in this situation, the cure rates can be high. These

---

TABLE 4.1

BCC: indications for Mohs' micrographic surgery

Site	**Size**
Eyelids	> 2 cm in diameter
Nose	
Nasolabial folds	**Other**
Ears, lips*	Recurrent BCC

Histology

Morpheic

Infiltrative

Micronodular

Perineural spread

*Some authorities include these sites in their criteria.

lesions require prolonged freezing for 20–30 seconds before the freeze–thaw cycle is repeated. Such prolonged freeze–thaw cycles are associated with significant morbidity.

Radiotherapy has been used to treat cutaneous malignancies for many years. It can be an excellent option for those not wanting to undergo surgery, and has a 5-year cure rate of 91% for primary BCC and 90% for recurrent BCC. It is generally thought that radiotherapy is best used for primary nodular and solid BCC.

Topical 5-fluorouracil is not commonly used to treat BCC, but it can be valuable in the management of superficial BCC, particularly of the face.

Topical imiquimod 5% cream is licensed in the UK for the treatment of small superficial BCC.

Photodynamic therapy (PDT) is an evolving technique. Current evidence suggests that 5-ALA PDT may be a useful treatment for superficial BCC, although it is not currently licensed for this indication. MAL PDT has been shown to result in high response rates in both superficial and nodular BCC, including difficult-to-treat lesions, and is licensed for this indication in Europe and Australia.

Follow-up. Most patients are reviewed 3–6 months after treatment. For an uncomplicated BCC, ongoing specialist care is not required. However, patients are advised to see their family doctor annually so that any recurrence or a further tumor at another site can be detected.

In-situ squamous cell carcinoma (SCC). Treatments reflect the range of clinical disease encountered. Bowen's disease is the most common form of in-situ SCC and a number of acceptable treatments are available. There are few studies comparing the efficacy of different treatment options, but expert opinion holds that no single approach is best for all clinical situations.

The treatments discussed below all have similar recurrence rates. In addition, preliminary studies have shown laser therapy and topical imiquimod to be effective, and other treatments are in development.

It is not uncommon for Bowen's disease to develop on the lower leg (see Figure 3.36), which is a site of poor healing. If an elderly patient presents with a lower leg lesion, observation may be the most sensible first-line management option.

Cryotherapy is a useful tool in the treatment of Bowen's disease. However, it can be painful and healing may be prolonged. Although there is controversy over the technique, a single 30-second freeze–thaw cycle appears to be as effective as two 30-second freeze–thaw cycles. The single 15-second freeze–thaw cycle is generally considered to be inferior.

Curettage with electrosurgery usually results in a less severe wound than that produced by cryotherapy, and can also be an effective treatment for Bowen's disease, although studies report cure rates ranging from 27% to 98%. The reasons for this variability are not clear.

Surgical excision is often used, depending on the size and site of the lesion. Mohs' micrographic or excisional surgery is recommended for digital and subungual Bowen's disease.

Photodynamic therapy is an effective treatment for Bowen's disease, and appears to offer good cosmesis and limited adverse effects.

Topical 5-fluorouracil is usually applied once or twice daily to the in-situ SCC for between 1 week and 2 months. It is a useful treatment for extragenital Bowen's disease, and penile and anal intraepithelial neoplasia (see Figure 3.38).

Radiotherapy. Although radiotherapy boasts high cure rates, it is often not a first-line treatment because there can be complications with poor wound healing.

Follow-up. Of the in-situ SCC subtypes, perianal Bowen's disease has the highest recurrence rates. Patients require long-term specialist follow-up, because they are at risk of further in-situ SCC and invasive perianal SCC.

Invasive squamous cell carcinoma. It is necessary to extirpate invasive SCC completely because of its potential to metastasize. This neoplasm usually spreads initially to the local lymph nodes via the lymphatics. SCC also has a tendency to develop in-transit metastases: these are cutaneous tumors adjacent to, but not contiguous with, the primary SCC.

Factors associated with high-risk SCC include large size, recurrent tumor and poor differentiation, as well as development at sites such as non-sun-exposed regions, an ear, a lip, or an area of skin damage or inflammation (see Figures 3.39–3.41). Patients with high-risk neoplasms are ideally managed by a multidisciplinary team of dermatologists, cutaneous surgeons and oncologists.

Surgical excision is the treatment of choice for invasive SCC in most patients. It achieves good cure rates and enables the SCC to be fully characterized histopathologically and the adequacy of the treatment to be verified microscopically.

For a well-defined SCC less than 2 cm in diameter, an excision margin of 4 mm is sufficient and provides a 95% cure rate. A wider margin of 6 mm or more is required for high-risk SCC. This excision margin may be smaller if the SCC is excised with Mohs' micrographic surgery or if there is intraoperative histological examination of the specimen edges. A wider margin is required because a high-risk cutaneous SCC may have surrounding, microscopic, in-transit metastases that must be removed. In addition, larger tumors have a greater degree of microscopic tumor extension.

Mohs' micrographic surgery (see Figure 4.1) should be considered for high-risk and recurrent SCC, particularly tumors at sites where it is difficult to achieve adequate excision margins. With reportedly the best cure rates for high-risk SCC, this is probably the treatment of choice for this subgroup. Some Mohs' surgeons will excise a further safety margin after histological clearance to allow for unidentified in-transit neoplasia.

Curettage with electrosurgery should be restricted to the treatment of small (< 10 mm diameter), well-differentiated, primary SCC. High cure rates have been reported. With this technique, it is difficult to ascertain histologically whether the tumor has been removed completely, although saucerization will give reliable, oriented histology.

Radiotherapy achieves cure rates comparable with those achieved using other treatments. It is the first-line treatment for non-resectable tumors for which the morbidity from surgery is considered too high. Radiotherapy is not suitable when the tumor has indistinct margins.

Management of lymph-node disease. If local lymph nodes are enlarged, they should be sampled by fine-needle aspiration or excisional biopsy for histological assessment. Ideally, node-positive patients should be reviewed in a multidisciplinary setting. Metastatic lymph-node disease is usually treated with regional lymph-node dissection. There is no strong evidence to favor prophylactic, elective lymph-node dissection, but it is sometimes performed for very deep SCC.

Follow-up. The patient with a treated high-risk invasive SCC is best observed for 5 years. The specialist, family doctor or patient can perform the surveillance.

Melanoma. The definitive treatment of primary cutaneous melanoma (see Figures 3.46–3.47) is surgical excision. After the diagnosis has been confirmed by excisional biopsy, surgical re-excision is usually performed.

Surgical excision. The rationale for removing a portion of normal skin surrounding the visible lesion is to prevent local recurrence. Melanoma cells have the capacity to migrate locally from the original tumor. Recommendations for the width of margins for surgical excision based on the Breslow thickness of the melanoma are presented in Table 4.2.

The margins should be measured clinically at the time of surgery and should not be imposed retrospectively following the histology report on the margin of excision, nor used to justify, erroneously, further surgery. There are circumstances in which the recommended margins may not be technically achievable or cosmetically or functionally desirable. If there is already evidence of metastatic disease, radical re-excision is illogical.

The treatment of lentigo maligna melanoma may be difficult because the margins can be clinically and histologically indeterminate (see Figure 3.44). As a minimum, the *nodular*

TABLE 4.2

Excision margins for primary melanoma

Breslow thickness of melanoma	BAD guideline margins	AAD guideline margins
Lentigo maligna and in-situ melanoma	2–5 mm to achieve complete excision	5 mm
< 1 mm	1 cm*	1 cm
1–2 mm	1–2 cm	1 cm
2–4 mm	2–3 cm (preferably 2 cm)	2 cm
> 4 mm	2–3 cm	2 cm

*Narrower margins are probably safe in melanoma with Breslow thickness < 0.75 mm.
BAD, British Association of Dermatologists; AAD, American Academy of Dermatology.

component of the lentigo maligna melanoma should be excised with the recommended margins.

The definitive approach for malignant melanoma with Breslow thickness less than 1 mm is contentious (see Figure 3.45). Many specialists excise these lesions with a narrower margin – there is no evidence of an adverse effect on prognosis when such lesions are excised with a margin of less than 1 cm, provided that the lesion has been unequivocally completely excised, as shown by histology.

Management of lymph-node disease. If there is clinical or radiological suspicion of lymph-node involvement, then fine-needle aspiration of the relevant nodes is recommended. It may be necessary to perform an open biopsy if there is persistent lymphadenopathy and fine-needle aspiration is negative.

Lymph-node metastases are treated with radical lymph-node dissection. Elective lymph-node dissection has not been shown to be advantageous for patients where there is no evidence of nodal involvement.

Sentinel lymph-node biopsy. There is controversy over the role of intraoperative lymphatic mapping and sentinel lymph-node biopsy.

The technique was first described by Morton in 1992 and is usually performed at the time of the wider re-excision. The sentinel lymph node is the first node in the lymphatic basin that drains the primary melanoma. It is dissected after identification by lymphoscintography. If histological examination proves metastatic involvement of the sentinel lymph node, then the patient undergoes complete nodal dissection. At present, there is no evidence that this procedure is beneficial, so it is not generally recommended for routine use. Sentinel node biopsy is an acknowledged sensitive staging tool in stage II disease. Because there may be some morbidity with the procedure it is probably best performed within a clinical trial setting. Further trials are required to clarify the role of sentinel lymph-node biopsy.

Adjuvant therapy. Despite many studies, no adjuvant therapy has been proved to be of value in the management of malignant melanoma. Individuals with stage IIB disease or higher have an intermediate to high risk of melanoma recurrence. These patients should be referred to a multidisciplinary team or melanoma center, where it may be possible for them to enter a trial of adjuvant therapy.

Much research has focused on the use of interferons as an adjuvant therapy. Interferons are cytokines with antitumor properties. High-dose interferon α is used in the USA as adjuvant treatment for high-risk melanomas. A randomized trial performed by the Eastern Cooperative Oncology Group reported increased survival in patients with melanoma with regional lymph-node spread or Breslow thickness greater than 4 mm who received high-dose interferon α2b compared with the control group. However, there was significant interferon toxicity and the results were not reproducible in a larger follow-up study.

The value of melanoma vaccines remains uncertain. Adjuvant limb perfusion has not been shown to be beneficial, but it may have a role in preoperative reduction of tumor volume.

Management of metastatic disease. At present, there is no treatment known to prolong survival significantly in patients with metastatic disease. Single local or regional metastases are treated by

> **Key points – management**
>
> - Excisional surgery is the gold standard for the treatment of most established skin cancers.
> - Cryotherapy is the gold standard for the treatment of actinic keratosis.
> - Traditional (5-fluorouracil) and modern (diclofenac and imiquimod) topical applications are popular alternatives for the treatment of actinic keratosis.
> - Mohs' micrographic surgery is the gold standard for selected BCCs.

surgical excision. Patients with multiple local metastases are best managed by a center specializing in regional therapies; patients may be offered chemotherapeutic limb infusion, interferon limb perfusion or carbon dioxide laser ablation.

Distant metastases at three or fewer sites should be considered for surgery. Dacarbazine remains the chemotherapeutic agent of choice for unresectable metastases. Palliative radiotherapy may be of value.

Follow-up. There is no evidence to justify a specific follow-up interval, but the consensus is to follow patients for 5 years. The US guidelines sensibly suggest that follow-up be determined on a case-by-case basis with reference to individual factors that include:
- Breslow thickness
- number of melanomas
- presence and number of atypical nevi
- family history
- anxiety
- patient capability.

British guidelines recommend that patients with invasive melanoma be followed up at 3-monthly intervals for the first 3 years; if the Breslow thickness is greater than 1 mm, follow-up should continue at 6-monthly intervals for a further 2 years. In many patients with stage I disease, the need for follow-up is dictated more by the patient's risk of having a second melanoma than by the risk of relapse from the original.

At follow-up, symptoms should be sought, the scar and the rest of the skin examined, and lymphadenopathy and organomegaly excluded clinically. Patient self-examination should be encouraged. Investigations are not necessary unless clinically indicated.

Key references

Ahmed I, Berth-Jones J. Imiquimod: a novel treatment for lentigo maligna. *Br J Dermatol* 2000; 143:843–5.

Bunker CB. Scientific evidence and expert clinical opinion for the investigation and management of stage I malignant melanoma. In: MacKie RM, Murray D, Rosin RD et al, eds. *The Effective Management of Malignant Melanoma*. London: Aesculapius Medical Press, 2001: 37–44.

Cox NH, Eedy DJ, Morton CA. Guidelines for management of Bowen's disease. *Br J Dermatol* 1999;141:633–41.

DeDavid M, Orlow SJ, Provost N et al. A study of large congenital melanocytic nevi and associated malignant melanomas: review of cases in the New York University Registry and the world literature. *J Am Acad Dermatol* 1997;36: 409–16.

Fritsch C, Goerz G, Ruzicka T. Photodynamic therapy in dermatology. *Arch Dermatol* 1998;134:207–14.

Gaspar ZS, Dawber RPR. Treatment of lentigo maligna. *Australas J Dermatol* 1997;38:1–8.

Geisse JK, Rich P, Pandya A et al. Imiquimod 5% cream for the treatment of superficial basal cell carcinoma: a double-blind, randomized, vehicle-controlled study. *J Am Acad Dermatol* 2002;47:390–8.

Graham GF. Cryosurgery in the management of cutaneous malignancies. *Clin Dermatol* 2001;19:321–7.

Morton CA, Brown SB, Collins S et al. Guidelines for topical photodynamic therapy: report of a workshop of the British Photodermatology Group. *Br J Dermatol* 2002:146:552–67.

Motley R, Kersey P, Lawrence C. Multiprofessional guidelines for the management of the patient with primary cutaneous squamous cell carcinoma. *Br J Dermatol* 2002;146:18–25.

Roberts DLL, Anstey AV, Barlow RJ et al. UK guidelines for the management of cutaneous melanoma. *Br J Dermatol* 2002; 146:7–17.

Sheridan AT, Dawber RPR. Curettage, electrosurgery and skin cancer. *Australas J Dermatol* 2000;41:19–30.

Slade J, Marghoob AA, Salopek TG et al. Atypical mole syndrome: risk factor for cutaneous malignant melanoma and implications for management. *J Am Acad Dermatol* 1995;32:479–94.

Sober AJ, Chuang TY, Duvic M et al. Guidelines of care for primary cutaneous melanoma. *J Am Acad Dermatol* 2001;45:579–86.

Spittle MF. Radiotherapy and reactions to ionizing radiation. In: Champion RH, Burton JL, Burns DA, Breathnach SM, eds. *Rook/Wilkinson/Ebling: Textbook of Dermatology*, 6th edn. Oxford: Blackwell Science, 1998: 3565–71.

Stockfleth E, Meyer T, Benninghoff B et al. A randomized, double-blind, vehicle-controlled study to assess 5% imiquimod cream for the treatment of multiple actinic keratoses. *Arch Dermatol* 2002;138:1498–502.

Telfer NR, Colver GB, Bowers PW. Guidelines for the management of basal cell carcinoma. *Br J Dermatol* 1999;141:415–23.

Walker NP, Lawrence CM, Dawber RPR. Dermatological surgery. In: Champion RH, Burton JL, Burns DA, Breathnach SM, eds. Rook/Wilkinson/Ebling: *Textbook of Dermatology*, 6th edn. Oxford: Blackwell Science, 1998:3622–3.

Basal cell carcinoma

The patient with a treated, uncomplicated basal cell carcinoma (BCC) can expect an excellent outcome. Following appropriate treatment, the recurrence rate is less than 10%. Factors associated with a poor prognosis include:

- infiltrative, morpheic or basosquamous histological subtypes
- immunocompromised status
- large or recurrent BCC
- location on the ear, nose, nasolabial fold or eyelid.

The literature suggests that, of recurrent BCC, 33%, 50% and 66% reappear within 1, 2 and 3 years of treatment, respectively. In addition, once an individual has developed one BCC, they have a greater risk of developing further BCC than those with no history of this tumor.

BCC spreads slowly by direct extension of the primary tumor (Figure 5.1). The morbidity from this neoplasm is largely caused by the destruction of surrounding normal tissue. This neoplasm very rarely metastasizes. The BCCs that appear to have greatest metastatic potential are the deeply invasive, morpheic tumors on the face or scalp.

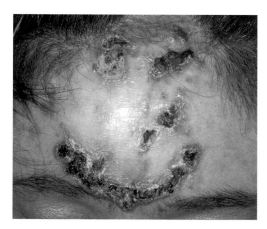

Figure 5.1 Recurrent BCC on the forehead.

Squamous cell carcinoma

In-situ squamous cell carcinoma (SCC). The recurrence rate following treatment for extragenital Bowen's disease is 5–10%. If left untreated, approximately 3% of extragenital in-situ SCCs will progress to invasive SCC, and the risk is higher with anogenital involvement.

An apparent relationship between Bowen's disease and internal malignancy was reported in the 1950s. A subsequent meta-analysis concluded that there was no significant association.

Invasive squamous cell carcinoma. If the invasive SCC is identified and treated early, the prognosis is better. The factors affecting tumor recurrence and metastatic potential are listed in Table 5.1.

Metastases are most likely to develop from larger, fast-growing, poorly-differentiated SCCs and those arising on high-risk sites. If the diameter of the SCC is greater than 20 mm, there is a 15% risk of recurrence and a 30% risk of metastasis. By comparison, the rates for smaller lesions are 7% and 9%, respectively. Neoplasms that extend into subcutaneous tissue and those with a depth greater than 4 mm also have a poor prognosis – 45% of these will metastasize.

TABLE 5.1

Risk factors for SCC recurrence and metastasis

Histological features	Location
Poorly differentiated	Lip
Perineural involvement	Ear
Dimensions	Non-sun-exposed sites
Diameter > 20 mm	Sites of scarring, Bowen's disease or inflammation
Depth > 4 mm	**Host factors**
	Immunosuppression

At the time of initial therapy, incompletely excised and recurrent SCC is more likely to metastasize than primary SCC.

The method of treatment influences the outcome. Recurrence rates following Mohs' micrographic surgery have been shown to be significantly lower than those seen in other treatment methods. One meta-analysis reported local recurrence rates of 3.1% with Mohs' micrographic surgery compared with 10.9% with non-Mohs' techniques, for primary SCC of the skin or lip.

Virtually all SCC recurrences and metastases occur within 5 years of initial therapy.

Melanoma

In-situ melanoma does not have metastatic potential, though there may be local recurrence. The recurrence rate of lentigo maligna treated with conventional excision is approximately 9%, whereas cure rates approach 100% with Mohs' micrographic surgery using rush permanent sections.

Of the known prognostic variables for melanoma, the Breslow thickness is the strongest predictor of survival. Why Breslow thickness is such a powerful prognostic factor is not known – it may be that it reflects tumor volume. However, the measurement is not precise, and human variability and error need to be taken into account. The prognosis with reference to the Breslow thickness is presented in Table 5.2.

TABLE 5.2

Melanoma: 5-year survival rates in relation to Breslow thickness

Breslow thickness	Survival
In-situ	95–100%
< 1 mm	95–100%
1–2 mm	80–96%
2–4 mm	60–75%
> 4 mm	50%

> **Key points – prognosis**
>
> - Basal cell carcinoma is a slow-growing tumor that very rarely metastasizes.
> - Approximately 3% of extragenital in-situ squamous cell carcinoma (SCC) will progress to invasive SCC.
> - SCC that is large, undifferentiated, recurrent or at a high-risk location is associated with a poorer prognosis.
> - Approximately 5% of lentigo maligna transform into lentigo maligna melanoma.
> - The Breslow thickness is the strongest prognostic factor for melanoma.

Other histological variables that adversely influence prognosis include:
- melanoma ulceration
- Clark's level of invasion
- numerous mitoses
- poor lymphocytic response
- tumor regression
- vascular invasion
- the presence of microsatellites.

Lesions located on the extremities have a better outcome than axial lesions, and there is a survival advantage for women and for patients under 50.

Neither pregnancy nor hormone replacement therapy has been shown to influence prognosis.

If the patient presents with melanoma and regional nodal metastasis, then the presence or absence of tumor ulceration has greater prognostic value than the Breslow thickness. In this group, the number of metastatic lymph nodes and the magnitude of tumor burden are also significant predictors of outcome.

Survival rates for melanoma stages I, II and III are shown in Table 5.3.

TABLE 5.3

Survival rates in primary tumor and regional lymph-node disease

Stage	Characteristics of primary tumor (including Breslow thickness)	Survival at 5 years
IA	≤ 1.0 mm, no ulceration	95%
IB	≤ 1.0 mm + ulceration	91%
	1.01–2.0 mm, no ulceration	89%
IIA	1.01–2.0 mm + ulceration	77%
	2.01–4.0 mm, no ulceration	79%
IIB	2.01–4.0 mm + ulceration	63%
	> 4.0 mm, no ulceration	67%
IIC	> 4.0 mm + ulceration	45%
IIIA	Any thickness, no ulceration and nodal micrometastases	67%
IIIB	Any thickness, ulceration and nodal micrometastases	52%
	Any thickness, no ulceration and ≤ 3 palpable nodes	54%
IIIC	Any thickness + ulceration and ≤ 3 palpable nodes	24%
	Any thickness + ulceration and ≥ 4 palpable nodes, matted nodes or nodes and in-transit metastases	24%
	Any thickness, no ulceration and ≥ 4 palpable nodes, matted nodes or nodes and in-transit metastases	28%

Lymphatic mapping and sentinel lymphadenectomy appear to have prognostic value in specific disease stages.

Although melanoma can metastasize widely, metastatic deposits most frequently occur in the skin (Figure 5.2), soft tissues, lung and liver. The 1-year survival rates depend on the site of the metastatic disease, as shown in Figure 5.3. In addition, elevated serum lactate dehydrogenase is associated with poor prognosis.

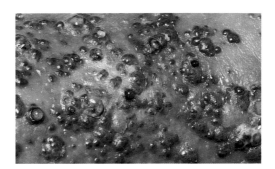

Figure 5.2 Cutaneous melanoma metastases.

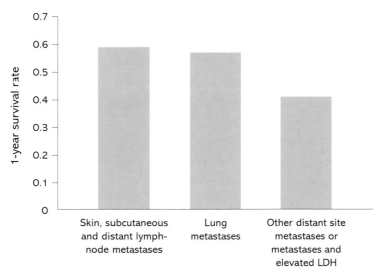

Figure 5.3 One-year survival rates for metastatic disease. LDH, lactate dehydrogenase.

Key references

Greene FL, Page DL, Fleming ID et al. Melanoma of the skin. In: *AJCC Cancer Staging Manual*, 6th edn. New York: Springer, 2002: 209–17.

Lang PG Jr. Malignant melanoma. *Med Clin North Am* 1998;82: 1325–58.

Rowe DE, Carroll RJ, Day CL. Prognostic factors for local recurrence, metastasis, and survival rates in squamous cell carcinoma of the skin, ear and lip. *J Am Acad Dermatol* 1992;26:976–90.

Exposure to UV radiation is the strongest recognized risk factor for cutaneous malignancy. Therefore, sun protection strategies are fundamental in the prevention of skin cancer. High-risk individuals require education, self-examination and close observation so that an early diagnosis can be made.

Chemoprophylaxis has a role in very high-risk cases that develop recurrent non-melanoma skin cancer.

Protection from the sun

Taking protective measures from the sun limits the penetration of UV radiation into the skin, minimizing the risk of photo-carcinogenesis, photoimmunosuppression and photoaging. Protection against UV light involves avoiding the sun, wearing protective clothing and using sunscreens.

Sun avoidance. Exposure to UV irradiation can be significantly reduced by avoiding the midday sun. The intensity of the UV light varies considerably throughout the day, with approximately two-thirds of all UVB and half of UVA radiation reaching the earth between 11 AM and 3 PM. Furthermore, a greater percentage of body surface area is irradiated by sunlight in the middle of the day when the sun is overhead. During this period, 50% of UVB still reaches shaded areas.

Sunscreens are topically applied lotions or creams that attenuate UV radiation. They can work in two ways:
• reflection of UV light by molecular scattering
• absorption of UV light by the cream and re-emittance as heat.
Sunscreens with a high sun protection factor (SPF) have only been available since the 1980s.

To be effective, sunscreens must remain on the skin in sufficient quantities throughout the period of sun exposure. Studies on the use of sunscreens by the public show that preparations are generally applied inadequately, with individuals repeatedly using less than the recommended amount. However, when they are used properly, sunscreens appear to be safe and effective.

The efficacy of a sunscreen is primarily assessed by the SPF, a measurement that quantifies the degree of protection provided from the erythemogenic wavelengths, which are primarily UVB. The SPF value is obtained after dividing the minimal erythema dose in sunscreen-protected skin by the minimal erythema dose in non-sunscreen-protected skin.

For non-melanoma skin cancer, the relationship between UVB radiation and photocarcinogenesis is well recognized. However, there is still uncertainty regarding the role of UVA, and the UV wavelengths involved in melanoma are unknown. Although more recently available sunscreens offer UVA and UVB protection, a standardized measure of UVA protection has yet to be elucidated. The American Academy of Dermatology (AAD) recommends using a sunscreen with both UVA and UVB protection, and with an SPF of 15 or higher.

In vitro, sunscreens have been shown to prevent photo-immunosuppression and the formation of UV-radiation-induced pyrimidine dimers and sunburn cells (keratinocytes undergoing apoptosis as a result of UV radiation). Studies have demonstrated that regular application of sunscreen prevents the development of actinic keratoses. Careful regular sunscreen use has also been shown to reduce the occurrence of SCC. One study showed that the regular application of SPF 15+ sunscreen for the first 18 years of life significantly reduced the lifetime risk of non-melanoma skin cancer.

Whether sunscreens can reduce the risk of melanoma has not yet been proven. Epidemiological studies have provided conflicting results and contain many inadequacies. For example, a common bias is seen with individuals who frequently apply sunscreens as they also tend to have a greater degree of sun exposure. It is difficult and probably unethical to perform a reliable study. In Australia there has been a reduction in the incidence of melanoma, and, as sunscreens are the most commonly used method of sun protection there, they are likely to be a major factor in this decline.

Protective clothing. Clothing often has an SPF of 20 or more and tends to absorb the spectrum of solar irradiation uniformly. Fabrics with a tight weave, a dark color and a heavy weight are more protective.

Wetness also alters the degree of protection; for example, a white, cotton t-shirt provides protection of approximately SPF 6 when dry and SPF 3 when wet.

As individuals are most commonly standing upright when exposed to sunlight, the sites of greatest irradiation include the scalp, face, upper back, forearms and hands.

A wide-brimmed hat is particularly protective; wearing a hat with a 10-cm brim has been shown to lower the lifetime rate of skin cancer significantly.

Skin-cancer prevention campaigns. The combined photoprotective approach of avoiding the sun, wearing appropriate clothing and using regular broad-spectrum high SPF sunscreen is currently the evidence-based recommendation of the AAD. This approach has been shown to reduce the incidence of non-melanoma skin cancer and appears to be reducing the incidence of melanoma.

In Australia, evidence suggests that the incidence of skin cancer is decreasing in people under the age of 50, who have been exposed to long-running sun protection messages such as the 'slip, slop, slap' (slip on a shirt, slop on sunscreen, slap on a hat) campaign. A similar message is now being promoted in the UK, with the launch of the SunSmart campaign in 2003, commissioned by the UK Health Departments and run by Cancer Research UK. The campaign focuses on the SunSmart message:

- Stay in the shade between 11 AM and 3 PM
- Make sure you never burn
- Always cover up
- Remember to take extra care of children
- Then use factor 15+ sunscreen.

Chemoprophylaxis

In patients developing recurrent non-melanoma skin cancer, chemoprophylaxis may be suitable and valuable. The administration of systemic retinoids as first-line chemoprophylactic treatment is an area of much research. Retinoids exhibit antineoplastic properties and are thought to work by binding nuclear receptors that enhance gene expression for cell differentiation and growth regulation. They tend to be offered to high-risk individuals, such as organ transplant recipients and patients with xeroderma pigmentosum or basal-cell nevus syndrome.

There is evidence that acitretin, 0.3 mg/kg/day, significantly reduces the development of non-melanoma skin cancers in renal transplant recipients who have previously developed SCC or BCC. Study participants have received acitretin for up to 5 years. Continuous treatment is required to maintain the protective effect; the benefit is quickly lost after the retinoid is discontinued.

Key points – prevention

- Protective measures against ultraviolet (UV) radiation involve wearing appropriate clothing, avoiding the sun and using sunscreens.
- UV radiation is greatest between the hours of 11 AM and 3 PM.
- Recommended sunscreens have both UVA and UVB protection, with an SPF of 15 or greater.
- Regular application of sunscreen in childhood has been shown to reduce the lifetime risk of non-melanoma skin cancer.
- Oral retinoid prophylaxis can be offered to very high-risk individuals to reduce the development of non-melanoma skin cancer.

Key references

Bastuji-Garin S, Diepgen TL. Cutaneous malignant melanoma, sun exposure, and sunscreen use: epidemiological evidence. *Br J Dermatol* 2002;146(suppl 61): 24–30.

Lim HW, Naylor M, Honigsmann H et al. American Academy of Dermatology Consensus Conference on UVA protection of sunscreens: summary and recommendations. *J Am Acad Dermatol* 2001;44:505–8.

Mahroos MA, Yaar M, Phillips TJ et al. Effect of sunscreen application on UV-induced thymine dimers. *Arch Dermatol* 2002;138:1480–5.

McKenna DB, Murphy GM. Skin cancer chemoprophylaxis in renal transplant recipients: 5 years of experience using low-dose acitretin. *Br J Dermatol* 1999;140:656–60.

Naylor MF, Boyd A, Smith DW et al. High sun protection factor sunscreens in the suppression of actinic neoplasia. *Arch Dermatol* 1995;131:170–5.

Rigel DS. Photoprotection: a 21st century perspective. *Br J Dermatol* 2002;146(suppl 61):34–7.

Thompson SC, Jolley D, Marks R. Reduction of solar keratoses by regular sunscreen use. *N Engl J Med* 1993;329:1147–51.

Urbach F. The cumulative effects of ultraviolet radiation on the skin: photocarcinogenesis. In: Hawk JLM, ed. *Photodermatology*. London: Arnold, 1999:99–100.

This is a pivotal time in the history of skin cancer and its therapies. The incidence of both non-melanoma skin cancer and melanoma has risen greatly over the past century – more than twentyfold in the case of melanoma – and continues to increase at an alarming rate. Although there is justified concern about the effects of the chemically induced thinning of the ozone layer, the increased numbers of people with skin cancer reflect, in large part, increases in and altered patterns of sun exposure in parts of the population. Changing dress and lifestyles, increased leisure time, the popular convictions that sun exposure is healthy and a tan is attractive, greater longevity and the affordability of distant travel to sunny climes have conspired to put a greater skin surface area at far higher risk from early adulthood into advanced old age.

'Safe sun' campaigns. Only after an unfortunate lag of 30–40 years has research progressively documented the central role of UV radiation in skin carcinogenesis. The causal relationship between UV radiation and skin cancer is corroborated by cellular, molecular and animal studies, as well as by epidemiological data. Dissemination of this information has given rise to more widely and effectively used sunscreens and to public health 'safe sun' programs, such as the comprehensive campaign promoted in Australia, where the combination of high isolation, a fair-skinned population and an outdoor lifestyle has resulted in the highest incidence of skin cancer in the world. Such campaigns offer the possibility of reversing the decades-long trends in morbidity and mortality from non-melanoma skin cancer and melanoma. Thus, it appears that UV radiation, the most prevalent human carcinogen and contributor to more than half of all human malignancies, is on the threshold of simple behavioral control; if adopted widely, conventional sun avoidance and strategies to protect people from the sun are predicted to prevent an estimated 90% of non-melanoma skin cancers and two-thirds of melanomas in the 21st century. It will be fascinating to learn whether humans will exercise this option, for one can enjoy sunshine while being more than 95% protected from unwanted sequelae. This is in contrast to the use of tobacco products, probably the second most prevalent source of carcinogens in modern society.

'High-tech' approaches to skin-cancer prevention may also shift the present balance between carcinogenic tissue damage and recovery. For example, applying a bacteriophage-derived DNA-repair protein to skin before or soon after sun exposure has already been demonstrated to reduce subsequent photocarcinogenesis. It also appears that the skin's innate protective 'SOS' response to DNA damage can be stimulated by topical application of a DNA fragment that mimics the physiological damage signal, without requiring the otherwise obligatory initial damage. The fragment alters the transcription rate of key genes, increasing both melanogenesis (tanning) and the repair capacity for future UV-induced photoproducts, thus decreasing the risk of skin cancer.

Chemoprevention – the use of a medication to arrest cancer progression – in already substantially sun-damaged 'initiated' skin, is likely to become an important adjunct to the current approach of close observation with biopsy of suspect areas. The first and best-documented chemopreventatives are retinoids, compounds derived from vitamin A or their synthetic analogs. Administered either topically or orally, for example, all-*trans*-retinoic acid, can reduce the number of discrete new premalignant and malignant lesions on the skin or the oral and respiratory mucosae. Much effort is now being expended to harness this effect while minimizing the potential short- and long-term side effects. It has also been ascertained that prostaglandin metabolism is elevated in SCC as a result of overexpression of the enzyme cyclooxygenase (COX)-2, which is induced by UV. Orally administered COX-2 inhibitors, now used most commonly to treat arthritis, appear to be promising agents for the prevention of cancers of the skin and intestinal mucosa. Additionally, inhibitors of ornithine decarboxylase, an enzyme required for cellular proliferation, have been shown to prevent both UV- and chemically induced tumors, as have various natural substances found in green tea, grapes and other foodstuffs, at least in animal models.

Biological therapy. Our understanding of the molecular events leading to non-melanoma skin cancer and melanoma has increased greatly in recent years. Particularly well documented are the roles of:

- mutations of the tumor suppressor *p53* gene in SCC
- *PTCH* or *SMO* mutations in BCC, resulting in deregulation of basal cell proliferation
- loss of p16^{INK4a}, a protein that inhibits progression through the cell cycle in melanoma.

In the foreseeable future, our understanding of the complex checks and balances that govern normal skin maintenance, as well as our appreciation of the defining characteristics for malignant versus physiological cell behaviors, may see targeted medical therapy replacing today's surgical procedures. It is already well documented that such medical approaches eliminate actinic keratoses, the precursors of SCC known to harbor the same *p53* mutations as the frankly cancerous lesions. Both metabolic toxins and immunomodulators have proved effective in the treatment of actinic keratoses, and increasing evidence suggests that the same agents can safely replace conventional non-specific destruction of BCC and SCC at least. For example, one therapy for actinic keratoses, recently approved by the US Food and Drug Administration, takes advantage of subtle enzymatic differences between normal and malignant cells to target the latter. This allows for more selective tumor destruction than gross visual or even microscopic delineation of skin cancers by the surgeon – and it leaves no scar.

Other therapies eliminate skin cancer by affecting the cutaneous immune response, inducing cytokine synthesis and stimulating lymphocytes to attack the abnormal tumor cells. In the future, targeting new blood-vessel formation and hence depriving tumors of the nutrients they need, may provide another selective and non-scarring approach. So powerful are these biological approaches – and so preferable from the patient's perspective – that within a decade, excision of skin cancers may well become the therapy of last resort, particularly for patients concerned with the impact of treatment on their appearance. Even the vested interests and natural conservatism of the surgical profession seem unlikely to prevent this therapeutic revolution. However, concerns about 'missing cancer' are likely to slow and restrict the use of new therapies, at least initially, to non-melanoma skin cancer, because of the relatively low morbidity and mortality associated with delayed therapy in the event that topical medication fails to eradicate the lesion.

The future. In brief, our understanding of and approach to this most common, most readily diagnosed group of malignancies – skin cancer – have changed in the past century and are likely to change as dramatically in the current one. The ability to prevent most skin cancers is already ours. Anticipated advances in the area should allow medical therapy to replace surgery in many instances, greatly reducing the discomfort, disfigurement and social cost now associated with eradication of these malignancies.

Key references

Bissonette R, Bergeron A, Liu Y. Large surface photodynamic therapy with aminolevulinic acid: treatment of actinic keratoses and beyond. *J Drugs Dermatol* 2004;3 (suppl 1):S26–31.

De Graaf YG, Euvrard S, Bouwes Bavinck JN. Systemic and topical retinoids in the management of skin cancer in organ transplant recipients. *Dermatol Surg* 2004;30:656–61.

Gilchrest BA. Using DNA damage responses to prevent and treat skin cancers. *J Dermatol* 2004;31: 862–77.

Goukassian DA, Helms E, von Steeg H et al. Topical DNA oligonucleotide therapy reduces UV-induced mutations and photocarcinogenesis in hairless mice. *Proc Natl Acad Sci USA* 2004;101:3933–8.

Marmur ES, Schmults CD, Goldberg DJ. A review of laser and photodynamic therapy for the treatment of nonmelanoma skin cancer. *Dermatol Surg* 2004;30: 264–71.

Silapunt S, Goldberg LH, Alam M. Topical and light-based treatments for actinic keratoses. *Semin Cutan Med Surg* 2003;22:162–70.

Touma D, Yaar M, Whitehead S et al. A trial of short incubation, broad-area photodynamic therapy for facial actinic keratoses and diffuse photodamage. *Arch Dermatol* 2004;140:33–40.

Yarosh D, Klein J, O'Connor A et al. Effect of topically applied T4 endonuclease V in liposomes in skin cancer in xeroderma pigmentosum: a randomized study. *Lancet* 2001;357:926–69.

Useful addresses

American Academy of Dermatology
PO Box 4014, Schaumburg
IL 60168-4014
Tel: +1 847 330 0230
Fax: +1 847 330 0050
mrc@aad.org
www.aad.org (includes information
on the Coalition of Skin Diseases)

American Skin Association
346 Park Avenue South, 4th Floor
New York, NY 10010
Tel: +1 212 889 4858
Fax: +1 212 889 4959
info@americanskin.org
www.americanskin.org

British Association of
Dermatologists
4 Fitzroy Square
London W1T 5HQ
Tel: +44 (0)20 7383 0266
Fax: +44 (0)20 7388 5263
admin@bad.org.uk
www.bad.org.uk

CancerBACUP (UK)
3 Bath Place, Rivington Street
London EC2A 3JR
Tel: +44 (0)20 7696 9003
Helpline: 0808 800 1234
Fax: +44 (0)20 7696 9002
www.cancerbacup.org.uk

Cancer Research UK
PO Box 123, Lincoln's Inn Fields
London WC2A 3PX
Tel: +44 (0)20 7242 0200
Fax: +44 (0)20 7269 3100
www.cancerresearchuk.org

DermNet NZ (New Zealand)
www.dermnetnz.org

The Skin Cancer Foundation (USA)
245 5th Avenue Suite #1403
New York, NY 10016
Tel: 800 SKIN 490
Fax: +1 212 725 5751
info@skincancer.org
www.skincancer.org

Skin Cancer Information Network
MARCS (Melanoma and Related Skin
Cancers) Line Resource Centre (UK)
c/o Wessex Cancer Trust
Bellis House, 11 Westwood Road
Southampton SO17 1DL
Tel: +44 (0)1722 415071
marcsline@wessexcancer.org
www.wessexcancer.org

Skin Care Campaign (UK)
www.skincarecampaign.org

**Xeroderma Pigmentosum Society
(USA)**
437 Snydertown Road
Craryville, NY 1521
Tel/fax: +1 (518) 851 2612
xps@xps.org
www.xps.org

Index

References to photographs are given in italics

FAST FACTS

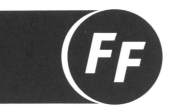

An outstandingly successful independent medical handbook series

Over one million copies sold

- Written by world experts
- Concise and practical
- Up to date
- Designed for ease of reading and reference
- Copiously illustrated with useful photographs, diagrams and charts

Our aim for *Fast Facts* is to be **the world's most respected medical handbook series**. Feedback on how to make titles even more useful is always welcome (feedback@fastfacts.com).

Fast Facts titles include

Acne
Allergic Rhinitis
Asthma
Benign Gynecological Disease (second edition)
Benign Prostatic Hyperplasia (fifth edition)
Bipolar Disorder
Bladder Cancer
Bleeding Disorders
Brain Tumors
Breast Cancer (third edition)
Celiac Disease
Chronic Obstructive Pulmonary Disease
Colorectal Cancer (second edition)
Contraception (second edition)
Dementia
Depression (second edition)
Disorders of the Hair and Scalp
Dyspepsia (second edition)
Eczema and Contact Dermatitis
Endometriosis (second edition)
Epilepsy (second edition)
Erectile Dysfunction (third edition)
Gynecological Oncology

Headaches (second edition)
Hyperlipidemia (third edition)
Hypertension (second edition)
Inflammatory Bowel Disease
Irritable Bowel Syndrome (second edition)
Menopause (second edition)
Minor Surgery
Multiple Sclerosis
Osteoporosis (fourth edition)
Parkinson's Disease
Prostate cancer (fourth edition)
Psoriasis (second edition)
Respiratory Tract Infection (second edition)
Rheumatoid Arthritis
Schizophrenia (second edition)
Sexual Dysfunction
Sexually Transmitted Infections
Smoking Cessation
Soft Tissue Rheumatology
Superficial Fungal Infections
Travel Medicine
Urinary Continence (second edition)
Urinary Stones

Orders

To order via the website, or to find regional distributors, please go to
www.fastfacts.com

For telephone orders, please call +44 (0)1752 202301 (Europe),
800 247 6553 (USA, toll free) or 419 281 1802 (Canada)